High Protein Vegetarian Gluten Free Dessert Cookbook

Over 100 oil-free, dairy-free, refined-sugar-free, low-carb Wholesome Treats for a Healthier You

Raimondi Hayden

ISBN: 9798876603791

DEDICATION
For as many who are ready to transform their dessert experience
without compromising on health

TABLE OF CONTENTS

INTRODUCTION

In the bustling chaos of modern life, I found myself yearning for a change that would bring both sweetness and wellness into my routine. Little did I know that a simple shift towards high-protein vegetarian, gluten-free, low-sugar, and oil-free dessert recipes would become the transformative force that reshaped my life

The journey began with skepticism, as the idea of indulging in desserts while prioritizing health seemed paradoxical. However, my taste buds soon met a revolution of flavors that defied expectations. Enter almond and chia seed energy bites, a revelation that not only satisfied my sweet tooth but also provided a sustained energy boost, thanks to the powerful combination of plant-based proteins.

Pistachio date bites followed suit, proving that decadence need not be sacrificed for nutrition. Rich in protein and free from gluten and excess sugars, these little delights became my guilt-free pleasure, showcasing the incredible synergy between wholesome ingredients. Avocado chocolate mousse became my go-to secret weapon for satisfying chocolate cravings without compromising nutritional goals. The creamy texture, enriched with the goodness of avocados, became a symbol of indulgence without regret.

As I embraced these high-protein, vegetarian, gluten-free, low-sugar, and oil-free creations, my body responded with newfound vitality. I witnessed increased energy levels, improved digestion, and a glow that radiated from the inside out. The scale might not have been the primary motivator, but it couldn't help but tip in my favor as a delightful side effect of this delicious lifestyle change.

Beyond the physical changes, my relationship with food underwent a profound transformation. Desserts were no longer mere treats; they became an essential part of my well-balanced, nourishing routine. The kitchen, once an intimidating domain, became my sanctuary for experimentation and creativity, proving that health-conscious choices need not compromise on taste.

Today, as I reflect on this sweet success story, I can confidently say that high-protein vegetarian, gluten-free, low-sugar, and oil-free desserts have not only tantalized my taste buds but have become the cornerstone of a life filled with health, happiness, and the unwavering belief that sweetness can indeed be a path to success.

High protein vegetarian desserts redefine indulgence by seamlessly blending sweet cravings with nutritional mindfulness. These desserts prioritize plant-based proteins, embrace gluten-free alternatives, use natural sweeteners, and achieve richness without excess oils. From protein-packed bites to chocolate innovations and fruit-focused creations, they offer a guilt-free and flavorful journey towards a healthier dessert experience.

Importance of Gluten-Free, Low Sugar, and Oil-Free Options

In today's wellness-focused culinary landscape, the emphasis on gluten-free, low sugar, and oil-free options extends beyond dietary preferences. These choices hold significant importance for various reasons:

1. **Dietary Inclusivity**: Gluten-free options cater to individuals with gluten sensitivities or celiac disease, fostering inclusivity in a diverse food landscape. Low sugar alternatives accommodate those managing blood sugar levels or seeking to reduce their overall sugar intake. Oil-free choices align with heart-healthy diets and cater to individuals aiming to minimize saturated fat consumption.

2. **Health-Conscious Living**: Gluten-free alternatives often utilize nutrient-dense flours like almond or coconut, contributing to a varied and well-rounded diet. Low sugar options support overall health by reducing the risk of diabetes, obesity, and other related health issues. Oil-free recipes promote heart health and help manage calorie intake, supporting weight management goals.

3. **Balanced Nutrition:** Gluten-free, low sugar, and oil-free options encourage a focus on whole, unprocessed ingredients, fostering a more balanced and nutritious diet. These choices often lead to increased consumption of fruits, vegetables, and plant-based proteins, contributing to a diverse nutrient profile.

4. **Digestive Wellness**: For individuals with gluten sensitivities or celiac disease, opting for gluten-free options can alleviate digestive discomfort and promote overall gut health. Reduced sugar intake supports digestive wellness by minimizing the risk of inflammation and maintaining a healthier gut microbiome. Oil-free choices can contribute to smoother digestion and absorption of nutrients.

5. **Weight Management**: Low sugar and oil-free options align with weight management goals, providing a satisfying culinary experience without excess calories. These choices often emphasize nutrient-dense ingredients, promoting satiety and reducing the likelihood of overconsumption.

6. **Adaptable to Various Lifestyles:** Gluten-free, low sugar, and oil-free options are adaptable to various dietary lifestyles, including vegetarian, vegan, and plant-based diets. They cater to a growing

demand for conscious and mindful eating, aligning with the preferences of individuals seeking holistic well-being.
The importance of gluten-free, low sugar, and oil-free options extends beyond dietary restrictions. These choices contribute to overall health, wellness, and a more inclusive, balanced approach to enjoying food.

Understanding the Ingredients

Navigating the realm of high-protein vegetarian desserts involves a keen understanding of key ingredients, each chosen for its unique role in crafting delicious and nutritious treats.

1. **Plant-Based Proteins:**
a) Sources: Legumes, beans, lentils, tofu, tempeh, nuts, seeds, and plant-based protein powders.
b) Role: Provides essential amino acids, promotes satiety, and contributes to muscle repair and growth.

2. **Gluten-Free Alternatives:**
a) Sources: Almond flour, coconut flour, quinoa, oats, and gluten-free baking blends.
b) Role: Accommodates gluten sensitivities, promotes a diverse nutrient intake, and contributes to a varied texture in desserts.

3. **Low Sugar Sweeteners:**
a) Sources: Dates, maple syrup, agave nectar, stevia, and monk fruit.
b) Role: Adds sweetness without the drawbacks of refined sugar, helping manage blood sugar levels and reducing the risk of related health issues.

4. **Oil-Free Cooking Techniques:**
a) Alternatives: Avocado, nut butters, applesauce, coconut milk, and yogurt.
b) Role: Enhances moisture and richness without relying on traditional cooking oils, aligning with heart-healthy choices and calorie-conscious diets.

5. **Whole Food Fats:**
a) Sources: Avocado, nuts (almonds, walnuts, pistachios), seeds (chia, flaxseed), and coconut.
b) Role: Contributes healthy fats, texture, and a rich flavor profile, promoting satiety and overall well-being.

6. **Natural Flavor Enhancers:**
a) Sources: Vanilla extract, cinnamon, nutmeg, and citrus zest.
b) Role: Elevates flavor without resorting to excess sugars or artificial additives, enhancing the overall sensory experience.

7. **Dairy Alternatives:**
a) Options: Almond milk, coconut milk, soy milk, and oat milk.
b) Role: Provides a base for creamy textures in desserts, accommodating lactose intolerance and aligning with plant-based lifestyles.

8. **Super-foods and Nutrient Boosters:**
a) Examples: Chia seeds, hemp seeds, spirulina, and cacao nibs.
b) Role: Augments nutritional content, adding antioxidants, omega-3 fatty acids, and other essential nutrients.
Understanding the role of each ingredient empowers the creation of high-protein vegetarian desserts that are not only delectable but also aligned with health and wellness goals. Aspiring dessert enthusiasts can experiment with these elements, embracing a culinary journey that celebrates both flavor and nourishment.

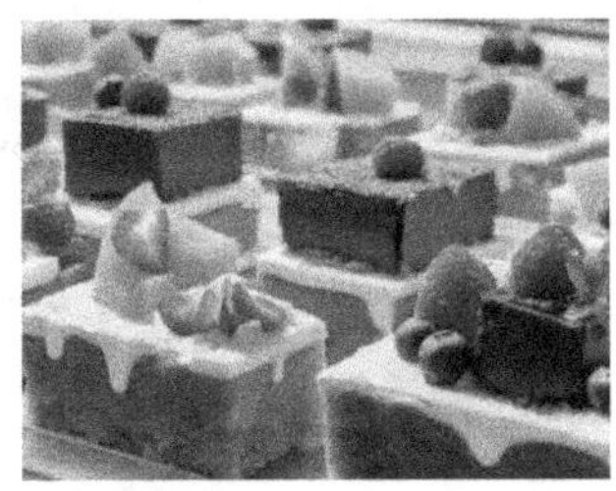

Storage and Shelf Life Considerations

Preserving the freshness and quality of high-protein vegetarian desserts involves mindful storage practices. Here are key considerations to ensure your delightful creations stay at their best:

1. **Refrigeration:** Many high-protein vegetarian desserts, especially those with perishable ingredients like tofu or dairy alternatives, benefit from refrigeration. This extends their shelf life and maintains optimal texture.

2. **Airtight Containers:** Store desserts in airtight containers to prevent exposure to air and moisture, which can lead to staleness or loss of quality. This is particularly important for items like protein balls, muffins, and bars.

3. **Freezing:** Certain desserts, like energy bites or muffins, can be frozen for longer shelf life. Ensure proper packaging to prevent freezer burn, and label containers with the date for easy tracking.

4. **Separate Layers:** When stacking or layering desserts, use parchment paper or silicone sheets to prevent sticking. This helps maintain the individual integrity of each piece and makes for a more visually appealing presentation.

5. **Fruit-Based Desserts:** Desserts with fresh fruits or fruit purees may have a shorter shelf life. Consume them within a few days or consider freezing to preserve their freshness.

6. **Nut and Seed Considerations:** Nuts and seeds, common ingredients in high-protein desserts, contain natural oils that can turn rancid over time. Store them in cool, dark places or the refrigerator to extend their freshness.

7. **Labeling:** Clearly label containers with the name of the dessert and the date of preparation. This practice helps monitor freshness and ensures you prioritize consuming items before their peak.

8. **Avoid Moisture:** Moisture can compromise the texture of desserts. Ensure that containers are completely dry before storing, especially for items like cookies or bars.

9. **Room Temperature Stability**: Some desserts, like energy balls or dried fruit snacks, are stable at room temperature for a short period. However, if they contain ingredients prone to spoilage, it's advisable to refrigerate.

10. **Check for Mold or Spoilage:** Regularly inspect stored desserts for any signs of mold, off odors, or changes in texture. Discard items that show signs of spoilage to prevent consumption of compromised food.

By incorporating these storage and shelf life considerations, you can enjoy high-protein vegetarian desserts at their finest, whether they are made for immediate consumption or saved for a later treat.

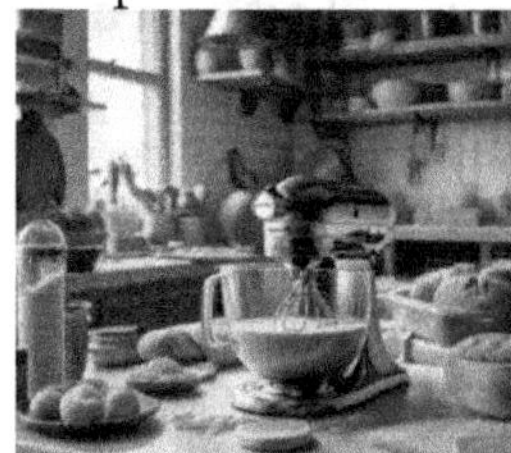

Balancing Flavors and Textures

Creating a delectable high-protein vegetarian dessert goes beyond meeting nutritional goals—it involves a delicate dance of flavors and textures. Achieving the perfect balance enhances the overall sensory experience. Here's how to master this art:

1. **Sweetness Harmony**: Utilize natural sweeteners like dates, maple syrup, or agave to impart sweetness without overwhelming the palate. Balance sweetness with tartness by incorporating citrus flavors, such as lemon or orange zest, to add complexity.

2. **Textural Variety:** Integrate a mix of crunchy and chewy elements. For example, combine nuts or seeds for crunch with dried fruits or oats for chewiness. Experiment with different textures like smooth and creamy (avocado chocolate mousse) alongside a crispy element (cacao nibs).

3. **Contrasting Temperatures:** Play with temperature variations for added interest. Serve warm desserts with a scoop of cold, non-dairy ice cream or chilled fruit compote for contrast.

4. **Layered Delight**: Consider building layers of flavors within a single dessert. For instance, a layered parfait with berries, yogurt, and granola offers a delightful interplay of tastes and textures.

5. **Savory Notes:** Infuse savory elements to balance sweetness. A pinch of sea salt in chocolate desserts enhances the richness, while spices like cinnamon or cardamom add depth.

6. **Fruit-Focused Brightness**: Fresh fruits not only contribute natural sweetness but also bring vibrant colors and refreshing flavors. Use fruits like berries or citrus to brighten up your desserts.

7. **Protein-Rich Binders:** Utilize protein-rich ingredients like nut butters, Greek yogurt, or silken tofu not just for nutrition but also for creating a creamy, luscious texture.

8. **Flour Alternatives:** Experiment with gluten-free flour alternatives to diversify textures. Almond flour may offer a denser, nutty texture, while coconut flour can add a lighter, fluffier element.

9. **Spice Elevation:** Incorporate warm spices like cinnamon, nutmeg, or ginger to add depth and warmth to your desserts. Spices contribute to a more sophisticated flavor profile.

10. Taste Testing: Regularly taste and adjust during the preparation process. Gradually add sweeteners or acids, such as lemon juice, and adjust textures until achieving the desired balance.

Achieving the perfect balance is a subjective journey. Tailor your high-protein vegetarian desserts to suit your personal preferences while considering the diverse palates of your audience. The art of balancing flavors and textures transforms your desserts into an extraordinary culinary experience.

Conclusion:

In the realm of high-protein vegetarian living, the journey is a delightful fusion of health-conscious choices and culinary exploration. By incorporating diverse plant-based proteins, balancing meals, and savoring protein-rich breakfasts and snacks, you open the door to a vibrant, flavorful lifestyle.

Experimenting with meatless days and relishing guilt-free high-protein vegetarian desserts adds a touch of culinary magic to your routine. Keep it simple with smart meal prep, explore global flavors, and let your body guide your protein choices.

In this journey, you're not alone. Connect with a community that shares your enthusiasm, exchanging ideas and experiences. As you savor the richness of a high-protein vegetarian lifestyle, may your days be filled with energy, satisfaction, and the joy of nourishing both body and soul. Cheers to a vibrant and delicious journey ahead!

Transformed breakfast recipes

These transformed breakfast recipes offer a delicious and protein-packed start to your day while adhering to vegetarian, gluten-free, low-sugar, and oil-free requirements. Adjustments can be made based on individual preferences and dietary needs. Enjoy your nutritious and satisfying breakfast!

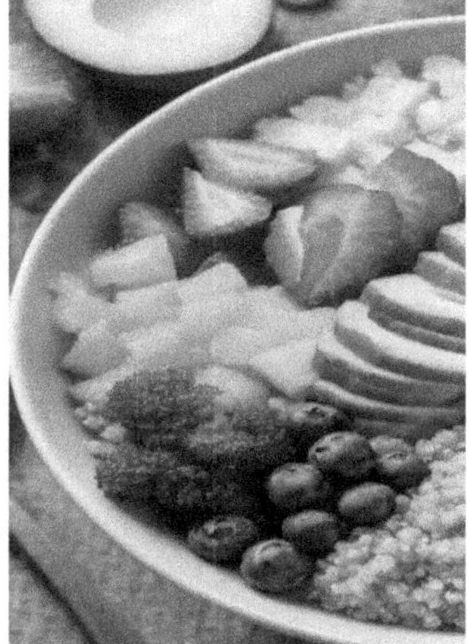

Quinoa Breakfast Bowl

A hearty and nutritious breakfast bowl featuring quinoa, fruits, and nuts.
Preparation Time: 15 minutes
Cooking Time: 15 minutes
Total Time: 30 minutes
Serving Size: 1 bowl
Ingredients:
1/2 cup cooked quinoa
1/4 cup Greek yogurt
1/2 cup mixed berries
1 tablespoon chopped almonds
1 tablespoon chia seeds
1 teaspoon honey or maple syrup
Directions:
1. In a bowl, combine cooked quinoa and Greek yogurt.
2. Top with mixed berries, chopped almonds, and chia seeds.
3. Drizzle with honey or maple syrup before serving.
Nutritional Info (per serving): Calories: 300 Protein: 15g Carbohydrate: 40g Fat: 10g Sodium: 40mg Potassium: 400mg Fiber: 8g

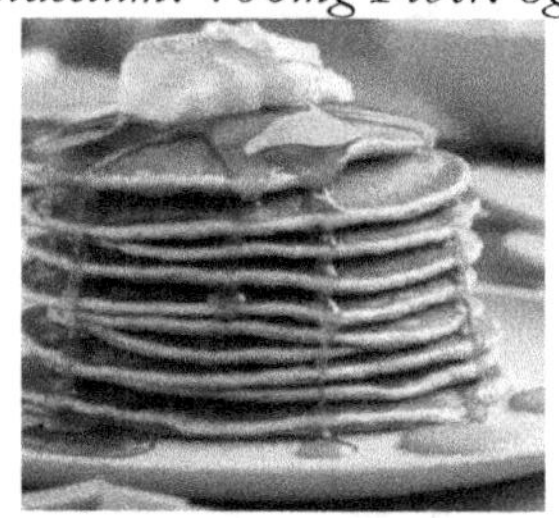

Sweet Potato Protein Pancakes

Fluffy and filling pancakes made with sweet potatoes and protein-rich ingredients.
Preparation Time: 20 minutes
Cooking Time: 10 minutes
Total Time: 30 minutes
Serving Size: 3 pancakes
Ingredients:
1/2 cup mashed sweet potato
1/4 cup oat flour (gluten-free)
1 scoop vanilla protein powder
1/2 teaspoon baking powder
1/2 cup almond milk

1 tablespoon maple syrup

Directions:

1. In a bowl, mix mashed sweet potato, oat flour, protein powder, and baking powder.

2. Add almond milk to achieve a pancake batter consistency.

3. Cook pancakes on a griddle and serve with maple syrup.

Nutritional Info (per serving): Calories: 320 Protein: 20g Carbohydrate: 40g Fat: 8g Sodium: 180mg Potassium: 350mg Fiber: 6g

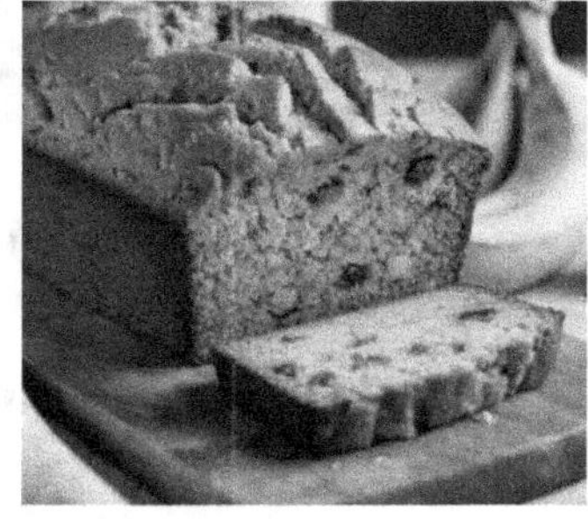

Almond Flour Banana Bread

A gluten-free and protein-rich twist on classic banana bread.

Preparation Time: 15 minutes

Cooking Time: 45 minutes

Total Time: 1 hour

Serving Size: 1 slice

Ingredients:

2 ripe bananas, mashed

2 cups almond flour

1/4 cup vanilla protein powder

1/4 cup almond milk

1/4 cup chopped walnuts

1 teaspoon baking soda

Directions:

1. Preheat the oven to 350°F (175°C).

2. In a bowl, combine mashed bananas, almond flour, protein powder, almond milk, chopped walnuts, and baking soda.

3. Pour into a greased loaf pan and bake for 45 minutes.

Nutritional Info (per serving): Calories: 280 Protein: 12g Carbohydrate: 20g Fat: 18g Sodium: 180mg Potassium: 320mg Fiber: 5g

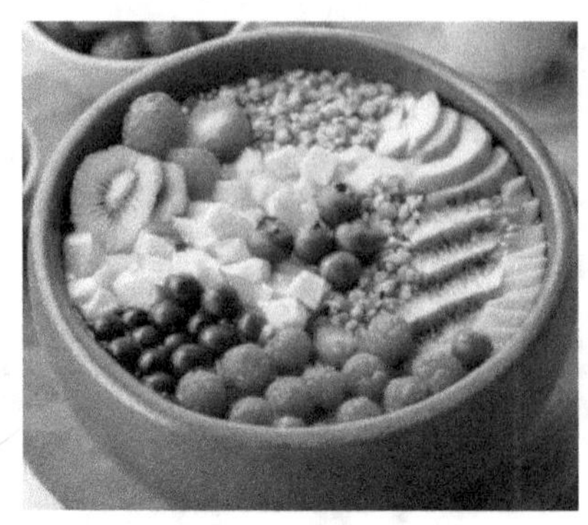

Protein-Packed Acai Bowl

A refreshing and energizing acai bowl loaded with protein and antioxidants.
Preparation Time: 10 minutes
Total Time: 10 minutes
Serving Size: 1 bowl
Ingredients:
1 packet frozen acai
1/2 cup frozen mixed berries
1/2 cup Greek yogurt
1 scoop vanilla protein powder
Toppings: sliced banana, granola, chia seeds
Directions:
1. Blend acai, frozen berries, Greek yogurt, and protein powder until smooth.
2. Pour into a bowl and top with banana slices, granola, and chia seeds.
Nutritional Info (per serving): Calories: 350 Protein: 25g Carbohydrate: 40g Fat: 10g Sodium: 60mg Potassium: 400mgFiber: 8g

Chickpea Flour Waffles

Crispy waffles made with chickpea flour, high in protein and fiber.
Preparation Time: 15 minutes
Cooking Time: 15 minutes
Total Time: 30 minutes
Serving Size: 2 waffles
Ingredients:
1 cup chickpea flour
1/2 teaspoon baking powder

1/2 cup almond milk
1 tablespoon apple cider vinegar
1 tablespoon ground flaxseed
Toppings: fresh berries, a drizzle of honey
Directions:
1. In a bowl, whisk together chickpea flour, baking powder, almond milk, apple cider vinegar, and ground flaxseed.
2. Cook the batter in a waffle maker until golden brown.
3. Top with fresh berries and a drizzle of honey.
Nutritional Info (per serving): Calories: 320 Protein: 18g Carbohydrate: 40g Fat: 10g Sodium: 380mg Potassium: 280mg Fiber: 8g

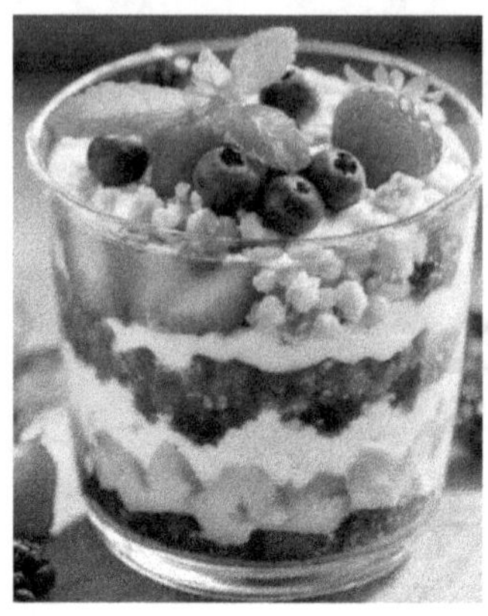

Cottage Cheese and Berry Parfait

A creamy and satisfying parfait with cottage cheese and fresh berries.
Preparation Time: 10 minutes
Total Time: 10 minutes
Serving Size: 1 parfait
Ingredients:
1/2 cup low-fat cottage cheese
1/2 cup mixed berries
1/4 cup granola (gluten-free)
1 tablespoon honey or agave syrup
1 tablespoon sliced almonds
Directions:
1. In a glass or bowl, layer cottage cheese, mixed berries, and granola.
2. Drizzle honey or agave syrup on top and garnish with sliced almonds.
Nutritional Info (per serving): Calories: 250 Protein: 15g Carbohydrate: 30g Fat: 8g Sodium: 300mg Potassium: 200mg Fiber: 4g

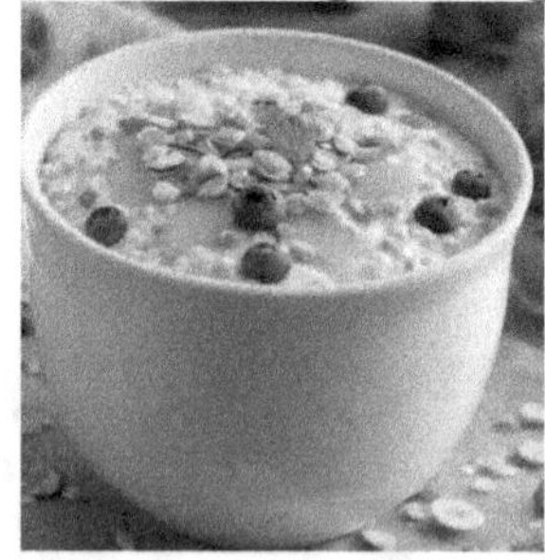

High-Protein Overnight Oats

A quick and nutritious breakfast with the convenience of overnight oats.
Preparation Time: 10 minutes
Total Time: 8 hours (overnight)
Serving Size: 1 bowl
Ingredients:
1/2 cup rolled oats (gluten-free)
1/2 cup almond milk
1/2 cup Greek yogurt
1 scoop chocolate protein powder
1 tablespoon chia seeds
Toppings: sliced banana, nuts, and a drizzle of nut butter
Directions:
1. In a jar, mix rolled oats, almond milk, Greek yogurt, protein powder, and chia seeds.
Refrigerate overnight.
2. Top with sliced banana, nuts, and a drizzle of nut butter before serving.
Nutritional Info (per serving): Calories: 380 Protein: 30g Carbohydrate: 40g Fat: 12g Sodium: 220mg Potassium: 400mg Fiber: 8g

Chia Seed Protein Pudding

A creamy chia seed pudding infused with protein for a delightful breakfast.
Preparation Time: 10 minutes
Total Time: 4 hours (chilling time)
Serving Size: 1 bowl
Ingredients:
2 tablespoons chia seeds
1/2 cup almond milk
1/2 cup vanilla Greek yogurt
1 scoop protein powder (vanilla)
Toppings: fresh fruit and a sprinkle of nuts
Directions:
1. In a bowl, whisk together chia seeds, almond milk, Greek yogurt, and protein powder.
2. Refrigerate the mixture for at least 4 hours or until set.
3. Top with fresh fruit and a sprinkle of nuts before serving.
Nutritional Info (per serving): Calories: 280 Protein: 20g Carbohydrate: 25g Fat: 12g Sodium: 150mg Potassium: 220mg Fiber: 8g

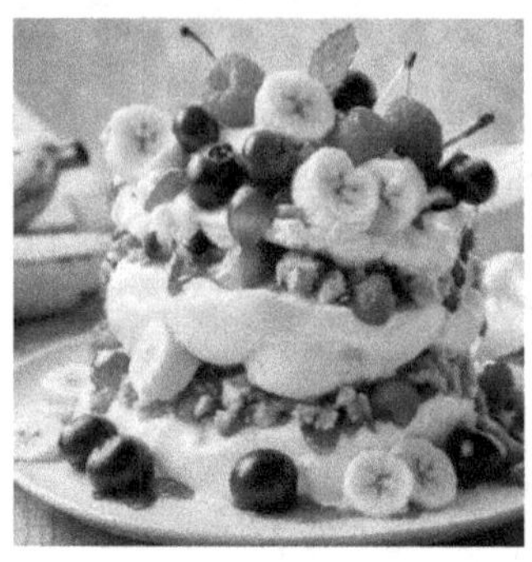

Protein-Packed Banana Split

A healthier version of the classic banana split with added protein.
 Preparation Time: 10 minutes
Total Time: 10 minutes
Serving Size: 1 banana split
Ingredients:
1 ripe banana, halved
1/2 cup Greek yogurt
1 scoop chocolate protein powder
Fresh strawberries, sliced
1 tablespoon chopped nuts
1 tablespoon dark chocolate chips (optional)
Directions:
1. In a bowl, mix Greek yogurt and chocolate protein powder.
2. Place banana halves on a plate, spoon the protein yogurt mixture over the banana.
3. Top with sliced strawberries, chopped nuts, and dark chocolate chips if desired.
Nutritional Info (per serving): Calories: 320 Protein: 25g Carbohydrate: 40g Fat: 10g Sodium: 120mg Potassium: 450mg Fiber: 6g

You will enjoy these sweetened-with-natural-goodness, high-protein, vegetarian, gluten-free, low-sugar, and oil-free dessert recipes

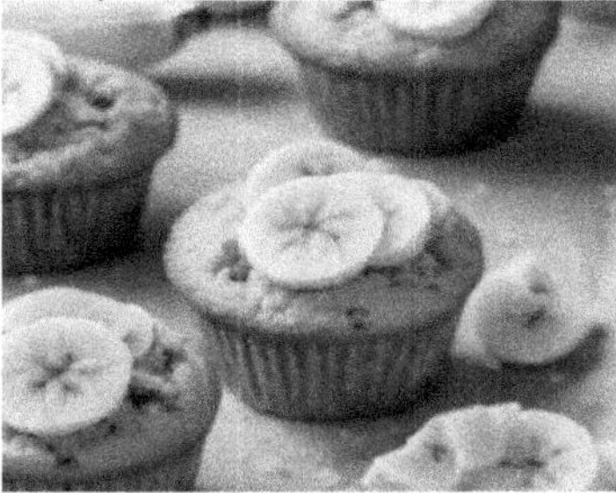

Blissful Banana Protein Muffins

Indulge in the perfect balance of sweetness and protein with these Blissful Banana Protein Muffins. They're gluten-free, low in sugar, and oil-free, making them a guilt-free treat for any time of the day.

Preparation Time: 15 minutes
Cooking Time: 20 minutes
Total Time: 35 minutes
Serving Size: 12 muffins

Ingredients:
2 ripe bananas, mashed
1 cup almond flour
1/2 cup vanilla protein powder
1/4 cup coconut flour
1 tsp baking powder
1/2 tsp baking soda
1/4 tsp salt
1/2 cup unsweetened almond milk
1/4 cup maple syrup
2 tsp vanilla extract
1/3 cup dairy-free chocolate chips (optional)

Directions:
1. Preheat the oven to 350°F (175°C) and line a muffin tin with paper liners.
2. In a large bowl, combine mashed bananas, almond flour, protein powder, coconut flour, baking powder, baking soda, and salt.

3. Add almond milk, maple syrup, and vanilla extract to the mixture, stirring until well combined.
If desired, fold in chocolate chips.
4. Spoon the batter into the muffin cups, filling each about two-thirds full.
5. Bake for 18-20 minutes or until a toothpick inserted comes out clean.
6. Allow muffins to cool in the tin for 5 minutes, then transfer to a wire rack.
Nutritional Information (per muffin): Calories: 120 Protein: 8g (27%) Carbohydrate: 12g (40%) Fat: 5g (33%) Sodium: 120mg Potassium: 180mg Fiber: 3g

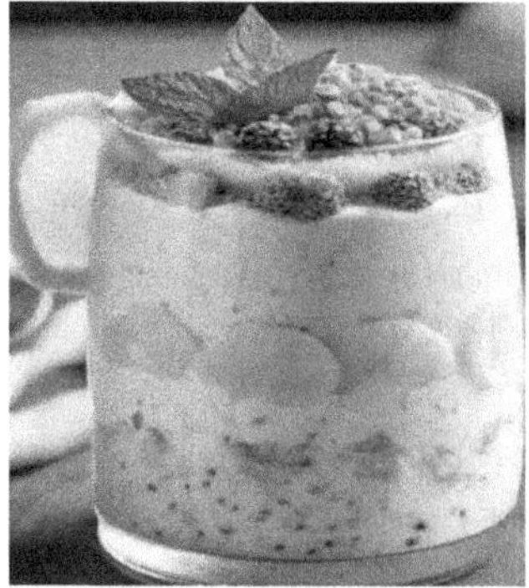

Luscious Lemon Chia Pudding Parfait

Savor the refreshing taste of citrus in this Luscious Lemon Chia Pudding Parfait. This gluten-free, low-sugar dessert is layered with wholesome ingredients for a delightful treat.

Preparation Time: 10 minutes (plus chilling time)
 Cooking Time: 0 minutes
 Total Time: 2 hours (chilling time included)
Serving Size: 2 parfaits

Ingredients:

1/4 cup chia seeds
1 cup unsweetened almond milk
1 tablespoon maple syrup
1 teaspoon lemon zest
2 tablespoons lemon juice
1 cup dairy-free yogurt (vanilla-flavored)
1 cup mixed berries (blueberries, strawberries, raspberries)

Directions:
1. In a bowl, combine chia seeds, almond milk, maple syrup, lemon zest, and lemon juice. Stir well and let it sit for 10 minutes, stirring occasionally.
3. 2. Cover the bowl and refrigerate for at least 2 hours or overnight, allowing the chia pudding to thicken.
4. Once the chia pudding has set, layer it with dairy-free yogurt and mixed berries in serving glasses or bowls. Repeat the layers until you get to the top.
5. Garnish with additional berries or a drizzle of maple syrup if desired.
Nutritional Information (per parfait): Calories: 250 Protein: 8g (13%) Carbohydrate: 30g (47%) Fat: 11g (40%) Sodium: 120mg Potassium: 300mg Fiber: 10g

Heavenly Chocolate Avocado Mousse

Satisfy your chocolate cravings guilt-free with this Heavenly Chocolate Avocado Mousse. Packed with natural goodness, this dessert is rich, creamy, and loaded with healthy fats.
Preparation Time: 15 minutes
 Cooking Time: 0 minutes
Total Time: 15 minutes
Serving Size: 4 servings
Ingredients:
2 ripe avocados, peeled and pitted
1/4 cup unsweetened cocoa powder
1/4 cup maple syrup
1 teaspoon vanilla extract
1/2 cup almond milk
Pinch of salt
Fresh berries for garnish
Directions:
1. In a blender or food processor, combine avocados, cocoa powder, maple syrup, vanilla extract, almond milk, and a pinch of salt.
2. Blend the mixture until smooth and creamy, scraping down the sides as needed.
3. Spoon the mousse into serving glasses or bowls.
4. Refrigerate for at least 1 hour to chill and set.
5. Before serving, garnish with fresh berries.

Nutritional Information (per serving): Calories: 180 Protein: 4g (9%) Carbohydrate: 20g (44%) Fat: 11g (47%) Sodium: 20mg Potassium: 480mg Fiber: 8g

Delightful Almond Butter Protein Bites

These Delightful Almond Butter Protein Bites are the perfect energy-boosting, gluten-free, and low-sugar snack. Packed with plant-based protein, these bites make for a guilt-free indulgence.

Preparation Time: 10 minutes
 Chilling Time: 30 minutes
 Total Time: 40 minutes
Serving Size: 15 bites

Ingredients:

1 cup rolled oats
1/2 cup almond butter
1/4 cup honey or maple syrup
1/4 cup vanilla protein powder
1/4 cup chopped almonds
1 teaspoon vanilla extract
Pinch of salt
Unsweetened shredded coconut for coating (optional)

Directions:

1. In a large bowl, combine rolled oats, almond butter, honey (or maple syrup), protein powder, chopped almonds, vanilla extract, and a pinch of salt, Mix until well combined.
2. Refrigerate the mixture for 10-15 minutes to make it easier to handle.
3. Roll the mixture into bite-sized balls, and if desired, roll each ball in shredded coconut for added flavor.
4. Place the bites on a parchment-lined tray and refrigerate for an additional 15-20 minutes to set.

Nutritional Information (per bite): Calories: 90 Protein: 4g (18%) Carbohydrate: 9g (40%) Fat: 5g (42%) Sodium: 20mg Potassium: 80mg Fiber: 1.5g

Raspberry Coconut Chia Seed Popsicles

Cool down with these refreshing Raspberry Coconut Chia Seed Popsicles. These gluten-free, low-sugar popsicles are not only a delightful treat but also a healthy way to beat the heat.

Preparation Time: 10 minutes (plus freezing time)

Freezing Time: 4-6 hours

 Total Time: 4-6 hours

 Serving Size: 6 popsicles

Ingredients:

1 cup fresh or frozen raspberries

1 can (14 oz) coconut milk

3 tablespoons chia seeds

2 tablespoons maple syrup or sweetener of choice

1 teaspoon vanilla extract

Directions:

1. In a blender, combine raspberries, coconut milk, chia seeds, agave nectar, and vanilla extract, Blend until smooth.

2. Pour the mixture into Popsicle molds.

3. Freeze for 1-2 hours, then insert Popsicle sticks into the partially frozen mixture.

4. Continue freezing for an additional 3-4 hours or until fully set.

5. Run the molds under warm water for easy removal.

Nutritional Information (per popsicle): Calories: 120 Protein: 2.5g (8%) Carbohydrate: 10g (30%) Fat: 8g (60%) Sodium: 10mg Potassium: 150mg Fiber: 4g

Nutty Quinoa Banana Bread

Indulge in the wholesome goodness of Nutty Quinoa Banana Bread, a gluten-free and protein-packed alternative to traditional banana bread. This recipe combines the sweetness of ripe bananas with the nuttiness of quinoa for a delightful treat.

Preparation Time: 15 minutes

Cooking Time: 50 minutes

Total Time:1 hour 5 minutes

Serving Size: 12 slices

Ingredients:

2 cups cooked quinoa, cooled

3 ripe bananas, mashed

1/2 cup almond flour

1/4 cup coconut flour

1/4 cup maple syrup

2 tablespoons chia seeds

1 teaspoon baking powder

1/2 teaspoon cinnamon

1/4 teaspoon salt

1/3 cup chopped walnuts (optional)

Directions:

1. Preheat the oven to 350°F (175°C) and grease a loaf pan.

2. In a large bowl, combine cooked quinoa, mashed bananas, almond flour, coconut flour, maple syrup, chia seeds, baking powder, cinnamon, and salt, mix until well combined.

3. Fold in chopped walnuts if desired.

4. Pour the batter into the prepared loaf pan.

5. Bake for 50-55 minutes or until a toothpick inserted into the center comes out clean.

6. Allow the banana bread to cool before slicing.

Nutritional Information (per slice): Calories: 150 Protein: 5g (13%) Carbohydrate: 23g (57%) Fat: 5g (30%) Sodium: 90mg Potassium: 250mg Fiber: 4g

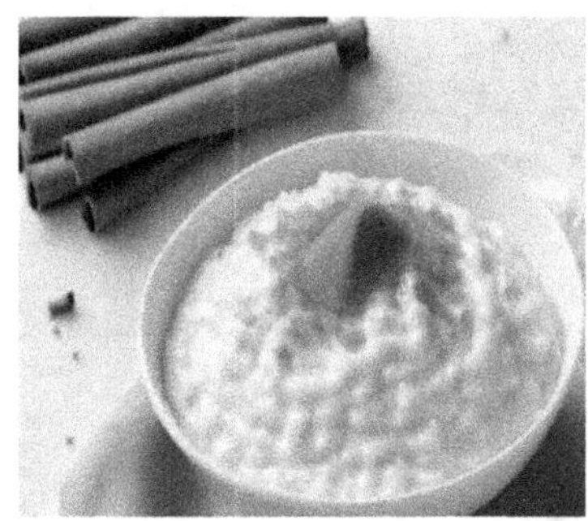

Vanilla Protein Rice Pudding with Cinnamon

Indulge in the comforting flavors of Vanilla Protein Rice Pudding with Cinnamon, a high-protein, gluten-free dessert. This creamy treat is sweetened naturally and offers a perfect balance of texture and warmth.

Preparation Time: 10 minutes
 Cooking Time: 25 minutes
Total Time: 35 minutes
 Serving Size: 6 servings

Ingredients:

1 cup jasmine rice, rinsed
2 cups unsweetened almond milk
1 scoop vanilla protein powder
1/4 cup maple syrup
1 teaspoon vanilla extract
1/2 teaspoon ground cinnamon
Pinch of salt
Sliced almonds for garnish (optional)

Directions:

1. In a medium saucepan, combine jasmine rice, almond milk, protein powder, maple syrup, vanilla extract, cinnamon, and a pinch of salt.
2. Bring to a boil, then reduce the heat to low, cover, and simmer for 20-25 minutes or until the rice is tender, stirring occasionally.
3. Once the rice pudding reaches a creamy consistency, remove from heat.
4. Allow it to cool for a few minutes, then stir before serving.
5. Garnish with sliced almonds if desired.

Nutritional Information (per serving): Calories: 180 Protein: 7g (16%) Carbohydrate: 35g (65%) Fat: 2g (19%) Sodium: 80mg Potassium: 120mg Fiber: 1.5g

Coconut Flour Carrot Cake Bites

Enjoy the taste of a classic carrot cake in a bite-sized, gluten-free form with these Coconut Flour Carrot Cake Bites. Packed with natural sweetness and a hint of coconut, these treats are perfect for guilt-free snacking.

Preparation Time: 20 minutes
Chilling Time: 30 minutes
Total Time: 50 minutes
Serving Size: 15 bites

Ingredients:

1 cup grated carrots
1/2 cup coconut flour
1/4 cup chopped dates
1/4 cup shredded coconut
1/4 cup crushed pineapple, drained
1/4 cup chopped walnuts
2 tablespoons maple syrup
1 teaspoon cinnamon
1/2 teaspoon nutmeg
Pinch of salt
Additional shredded coconut for coating (optional)

Directions:

1. In a food processor, combine grated carrots, coconut flour, chopped dates, shredded coconut, crushed pineapple, chopped walnuts, maple syrup, cinnamon, nutmeg, and a pinch of salt.
2. Pulse until the mixture forms a dough-like consistency.
3. Scoop out small portions and roll into bite-sized balls.
4. If desired, roll each bite in additional shredded coconut for added texture.
5. Place the bites on a parchment-lined tray and refrigerate for at least 30 minutes to set.

Nutritional Information (per bite): Calories: 70 Protein: 1.5g (9%) Carbohydrate: 10g (57%) Fat: 3g (34%) Sodium: 10mg Potassium: 80mg Fiber: 3g

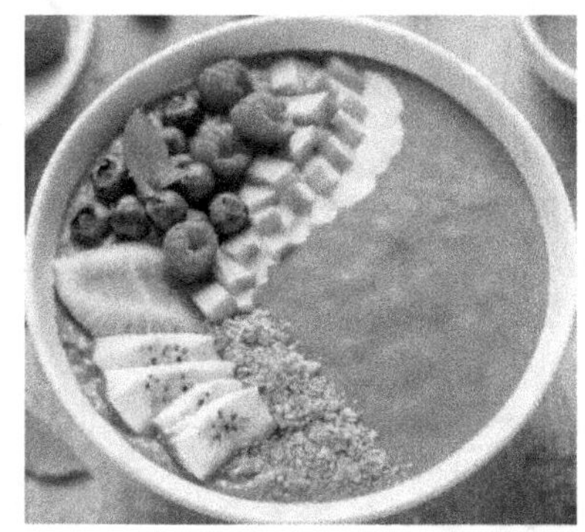

Matcha Green Tea Protein Smoothie Bowl

Elevate your dessert game with this refreshing Matcha Green Tea Protein Smoothie Bowl. Packed with antioxidants and protein, this gluten-free and low-sugar treat is not only delicious but also nutritious.

Preparation Time: 10 minutes
 Total Time: 10 minutes
Serving Size: 2 servings

Ingredients:

2 frozen bananas, sliced
1 cup spinach leaves
1 cup unsweetened almond milk
2 tablespoons vanilla protein powder
1 tablespoon chia seeds
1 teaspoon matcha green tea powder
1/2 teaspoon honey or agave nectar
Sliced kiwi, berries, and granola for topping

Directions:

1. In a blender, combine frozen bananas, spinach, almond milk, protein powder, chia seeds, matcha powder, and honey, Blend until smooth and creamy.
2. Pour the smoothie into bowls.
3. Top with sliced kiwi, berries, and a sprinkle of granola.
4. Serve immediately and enjoy with a spoon!

Nutritional Information (per serving): Calories: 220 Protein: 9g (16%) Carbohydrate: 40g (70%) Fat: 4g (14%) Sodium: 100mg Potassium: 550mg Fiber: 7g

Cacao Nib and Coconut Energy Bites

Energize your day with these Cacao Nib and Coconut Energy Bites. Packed with natural sweetness and the crunch of cacao nibs, these gluten-free, low-sugar bites are perfect for a quick and satisfying pick-me-up.

Preparation Time: 15 minutes
Chilling Time: 30 minutes
Total Time: 45 minutes
Serving Size: 12 bites

Ingredients:

1 cup pitted dates
1/2 cup almonds
1/4 cup cacao nibs
1/4 cup unsweetened shredded coconut
2 tablespoons chia seeds
1 tablespoon coconut oil, melted
1 teaspoon vanilla extract
Pinch of sea salt
Additional shredded coconut for rolling (optional)

Directions:

1. In a food processor, combine dates, almonds, cacao nibs, shredded coconut, chia seeds, melted coconut oil, vanilla extract, and a pinch of sea salt.
2. Pulse until the mixture reaches a dough-like consistency.
3. Scoop out small portions and roll into bite-sized balls.
4. If desired, roll each bite in additional shredded coconut for added texture.
5. Place the bites on a parchment-lined tray and refrigerate for at least 30 minutes to set.

Nutritional Information (per bite): Calories: 90 Protein: 2g (9%) Carbohydrate: 12g (57%) Fat: 4.5g (34%) Sodium: 5mg\ Potassium: 110mg Fiber: 3g

NO BAKE RECIPES

These recipes offer a variety of flavors and textures while ensuring they meet your criteria for high protein, vegetarian, gluten-free, low sugar, and oil-free desserts. You can make an Adjustments based on your personal preferences and dietary needs.

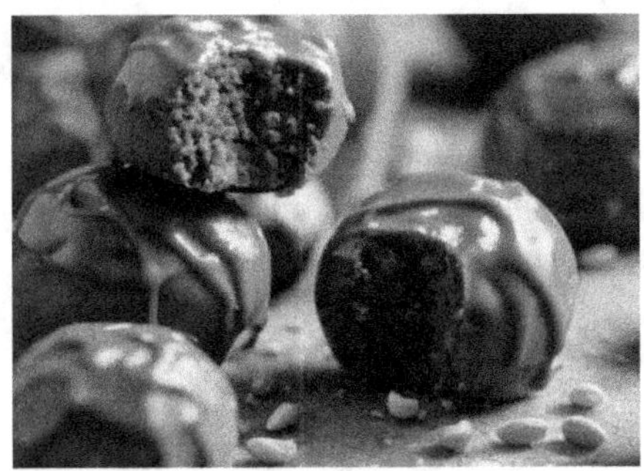

Chocolate Peanut Butter Protein Balls

These protein balls are a delicious combination of chocolate and peanut butter, packed with protein for a guilt-free treat.

Preparation Time: 15 minutes

Total Time: 1 hour

Serving Size: 2 balls

Ingredients:

1 cup rolled oats (gluten-free)

1/2 cup chocolate protein powder

1/2 cup natural peanut butter

1/4 cup honey or maple syrup

1/4 cup almond milk

1/4 cup dark chocolate chips (optional)

Directions:

1. In a bowl, mix oats, protein powder, peanut butter, honey, and almond milk.

2. Form the mixture into small balls and place on a tray.

3. Optional: Melt dark chocolate and drizzle over the balls.

4. Refrigerate for an hour before serving.

Nutritional Info (per serving): Calories: 180 Protein: 10g Carbohydrate: 18g Fat: 8g Sodium: 45mg Potassium: 200mg Fiber: 3g

Chocolate Almond Protein Bites

Satisfy your sweet tooth with these no-bake chocolate almond protein bites. Packed with protein and wholesome ingredients, they make a perfect guilt-free treat.

Preparation Time: 15 minutes

Total Time: 1 hour (chilling time included)

Serving Size: 2 bites

Ingredients:

1 cup almond flour
1/4 cup chocolate protein powder
2 tablespoons unsweetened cocoa powder
1/4 cup almond butter
2 tablespoons maple syrup
1 teaspoon vanilla extract
Pinch of sea salt
Unsweetened shredded coconut for rolling (optional)

Directions:

1. In a bowl, mix almond flour, chocolate protein powder, cocoa powder, almond butter, maple syrup, vanilla extract, and a pinch of sea salt until well combined.

2. Form the mixture into small bite-sized balls.

3. Optional: Roll the balls in unsweetened shredded coconut for an extra layer of flavor.

4. Place the bites on a tray and refrigerate for at least 1 hour to set.

5. Enjoy these delicious and protein-packed chocolate almond bites!

Nutritional Info (per serving - 2 bites): Calories: 160 Protein: 10g (25%) Carbohydrate: 10g (40%) Fat: 10g (35%) Sodium: 30mg Potassium: 120mg Fiber: 4g

Healthy Nuts Banana Protein Bars

These no-bake healthy nuts banana protein bars are a quick and easy snack, perfect for satisfying your cravings without the need for an oven.

Preparation Time: 15 minutes
Total Time: 1 hour (chilling time included)
Serving Size: 1 bar

Ingredients:

2 ripe bananas, mashed
1/2 cup peanut butter
1/4 cup vanilla protein powder
1 cup rolled oats
1/4 cup chopped nuts (walnuts, almonds, or as you want)

1 teaspoon cinnamon
Pinch of sea salt
Directions:
1. In a bowl, combine mashed bananas, peanut butter, vanilla protein powder, rolled oats, chopped nuts, cinnamon, and a pinch of sea salt.
2. Mix until well combined.
3. Press the mixture into a lined pan to create an even layer.
4. Refrigerate for at least 1 hour to set.
5. Cut into bars and enjoy these tasty and protein-rich peanut butter banana bars!
Nutritional Info (per serving - 1 bar): Calories: 220Protein: 12g (22%)Carbohydrate: 20g (35%) Fat: 11g (43%) Sodium: 70mg Potassium: 250mg Fiber: 4g

Coconut Chia Seed Pudding

Indulge in a creamy and satisfying coconut chia seed pudding, rich in protein and perfect for a quick and no-bake dessert.
Preparation Time: 10 minutes
Total Time: 4 hours (chilling time included)
Serving Size: 1/2 cup
Ingredients:
1/4 cup chia seeds
1 cup unsweetened coconut milk
1/4 cup vanilla protein powder
1 tablespoon shredded coconut (unsweetened)
1 tablespoon maple syrup (optional)
Fresh berries for topping
Directions:
1. In a bowl, whisk together chia seeds, coconut milk, vanilla protein powder, shredded coconut, and maple syrup (if using).
2. Let the mixture sit for 10 minutes, stirring occasionally to prevent clumping.
3. Refrigerate the mixture for at least 4 hours or overnight until it reaches a pudding-like consistency.
4. Top with fresh berries before serving.
5. Enjoy this creamy and protein-packed coconut chia seed pudding!

Nutritional Info (per serving - 1/2 cup): Calories: 180 Protein: 10g (22%) Carbohydrate: 14g (38%) Fat: 10g (40%) Sodium: 40mg Potassium: 130mg Fiber: 8g

Almond Joy Protein Balls

Savor the flavors of an Almond Joy with these no-bake protein balls. Packed with almond, coconut, and chocolate, they make for a delightful and energizing treat.
Preparation Time: 15 minutes
Total Time: 1 hour (chilling time included)
Serving Size: 2 balls
Ingredients:
1/2 cup almond flour
1/4 cup vanilla protein powder
2 tablespoons unsweetened shredded coconut
2 tablespoons almond butter
1 tablespoon maple syrup
1/4 cup dark chocolate chips (sugar-free)
Directions:
1. In a bowl, mix almond flour, vanilla protein powder, shredded coconut, almond butter, and maple syrup until well combined.
2. Fold in dark chocolate chips.
3. Form the mixture into small balls and place them on a tray.
4. Refrigerate for at least 1 hour to set.
5. Enjoy these Almond Joy-inspired protein balls!
Nutritional Info (per serving - 2 balls): Calories: 180 Protein: 10g (22%)Carbohydrate: 14g (38%)Fat: 12g (40%) Sodium: 20mg Potassium: 90mg Fiber: 4g

No-Bake Lemon Blueberry Cheesecake Bars

Indulge in the refreshing combination of lemon and blueberry with these no-bake cheesecake bars. High in protein and bursting with fruity flavors.
Preparation Time: 20 minutes
Total Time: 4 hours (chilling time included)
Serving Size: 1 bar
Ingredients:
1 cup cashews, soaked and drained
1/4 cup lemon juice
1/4 cup vanilla protein powder
2 tablespoons coconut flour

2 tablespoons maple syrup
1/2 cup fresh blueberries
Directions:
1. In a food processor, blend soaked cashews, lemon juice, vanilla protein powder, coconut flour, and maple syrup until smooth.
2. Line a pan with parchment paper and spread half of the mixture as the base.
3. Add a layer of fresh blueberries.
4. Spread the remaining cashew mixture on top.
5. Refrigerate for at least 4 hours to set.
6. Slice into bars and enjoy these luscious Lemon Blueberry Cheesecake Bars!

Nutritional Info (per serving - 1 bar): Calories: 220 Protein: 12g (22%) Carbohydrate: 18g (40%) Fat: 14g (38%) Sodium: 5mg Potassium: 230mg Fiber: 3g

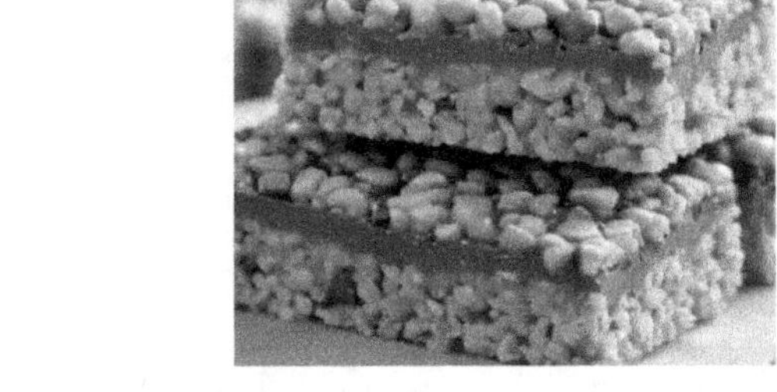

Chocolate Peanut Butter Rice Krispie Treats

Indulge in a childhood favorite with a protein twist. These no-bake Chocolate Peanut Butter Rice Krispie Treats are perfect for a quick and satisfying snack.
Preparation Time: 15 minutes
Total Time: 1 hour (chilling time included)
Serving Size: 1 square
Ingredients:
2 cups brown rice crisps
1/2 cup peanut butter
1/4 cup chocolate protein powder
2 tablespoons maple syrup
1/4 cup dark chocolate chips (sugar-free)
Directions:
1. In a large bowl, mix brown rice crisps with peanut butter, chocolate protein powder, and maple syrup until well coated.

2. Fold in dark chocolate chips.
3. Press the mixture into a lined pan to create an even layer.
4. Refrigerate for at least 1 hour to set.
5. Cut into squares and enjoy these delightful Chocolate Peanut Butter Rice Krispie Treats!
Nutritional Info (per serving - 1 square): Calories: 180 Protein: 8g (18%) Carbohydrate: 20g (44%) Fat: 8g (38%) Sodium: 50mg Potassium: 90mg Fiber: 3g

Chia Seed Pudding

A simple, creamy pudding rich in omega-3 fatty acids and protein.
Preparation Time: 10 minutes
Total Time: 4 hours (chilling time)
Serving Size: 1 cup
Ingredients:
1/4 cup chia seeds
1 cup almond milk
1 tsp vanilla extract
1 tbsp maple syrup
Fresh berries for topping
Directions:
1. Mix chia seeds, almond milk, vanilla extract, and maple syrup in a bowl.
2. Refrigerate for at least 4 hours or overnight.
3. Top with fresh berries before serving.
Nutritional Info (per serving): Calories: 180 Protein: 6g Carbohydrate: 22g Fat: 8g Sodium: 80mg Potassium: 120mg Fiber: 10g

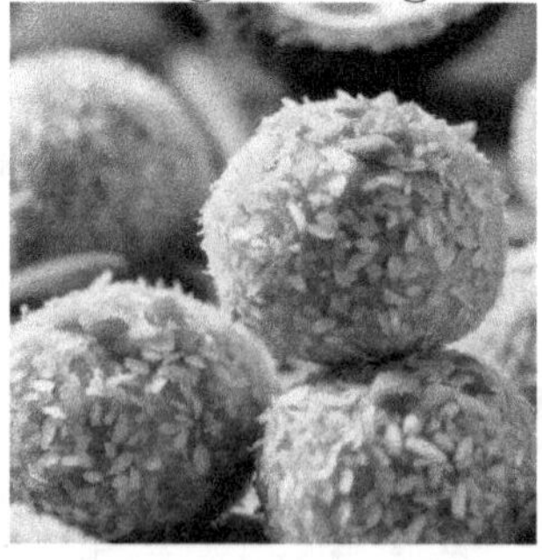

Coconut Almond Energy Bites

A tropical-flavored energy bite with the goodness of coconut and almonds.
Preparation Time: 20 minutes
Total Time: 1 hour
Serving Size: 2 bites
Ingredients:
1 cup shredded coconut (unsweetened)
1/2 cup almond flour
1/4 cup coconut flour
1/4 cup chopped almonds
2 tbsp maple syrup
1/4 cup coconut milk
Directions:
1. Combine shredded coconut, almond flour, coconut flour, and chopped almonds.
2. Add maple syrup and coconut milk, mix until well combined.
3. Form into bite-sized balls and refrigerate for an hour.
Nutritional Info (per serving): Calories: 160 Protein: 5g Carbohydrate: 14g Fat: 10g Sodium: 15mg Potassium: 180mg Fiber: 5g

Protein-Packed Berry Parfait

A refreshing and protein-rich parfait with mixed berries.
Preparation Time: 15 minutes
Total Time: 1 hour
Serving Size: 1 cup
Ingredients:
1 cup Greek yogurt (unsweetened)
1 scoop vanilla protein powder
1 cup mixed berries (strawberries, blueberries, raspberries)
1 tbsp honey or agave syrup
Granola for topping (optional)
Directions:
1. In a bowl, mix Greek yogurt and vanilla protein powder.
2. Layer the yogurt mixture with mixed berries in a glass.
3. Drizzle honey on top and garnish with granola if desired.
Nutritional Info (per serving): Calories: 220 Protein: 25g Carbohydrate: 20g Fat: 5g Sodium: 60mg Potassium: 280mg Fiber: 3g

No-Bake Quinoa Almond Bars

A crunchy and protein-packed bar with the goodness of quinoa and almonds.
Preparation Time: 20 minutes
Total Time: 2 hours
Serving Size: 1 bar
Ingredients:
1 cup cooked quinoa
1/2 cup almond butter
1/4 cup honey or agave syrup
1/4 cup chopped almonds
1/4 cup dried cranberries
1 tsp vanilla extract
Directions:
1. Mix cooked quinoa, almond butter, honey or agave syrup, chopped almonds, dried cranberries, and vanilla extract in a bowl.
2. Press the mixture into a lined pan and refrigerate for 2 hours.
3. Cut into bars before serving.
Nutritional Info (per serving): Calories: 180 Protein: 7g Carbohydrate: 20g Fat: 9g Sodium: 25mg Potassium: 150mg Fiber: 3g

Vanilla Almond Bliss Balls

Bliss balls with a hint of vanilla and the nutty goodness of almonds.
Preparation Time: 15 minutes
Total Time: 1 hour
Serving Size: 2 balls
Ingredients:
1 cup almond flour
1/4 cup vanilla protein powder
1/4 cup almond butter
2 tbsp unsweetened almond milk
1 tsp vanilla extract
Shredded coconut for rolling (optional)
Directions:
1. In a bowl, combine almond flour, vanilla protein powder, almond butter, almond milk, and vanilla extract.
2. Form the mixture into balls and roll them in shredded coconut if desired.
3. Refrigerate for an hour before serving.

Nutritional Info (per serving): Calories: 160 Protein: 8g Carbohydrate: 8g Fat: 10g Sodium: 20mg Potassium: 120mg Fiber: 4g

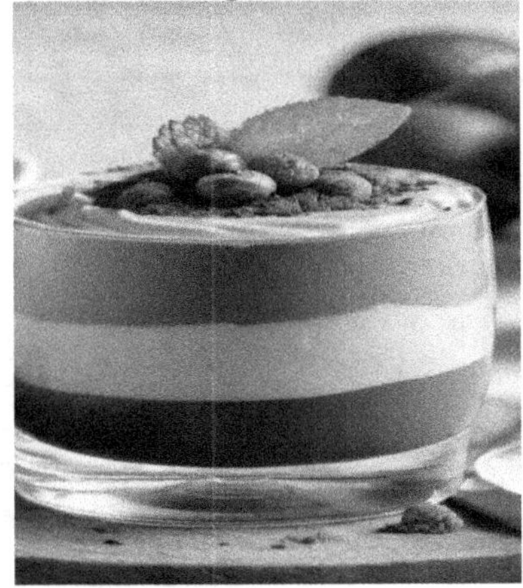

Avocado Chocolate Mousse

A creamy chocolate mousse made with the healthy fats of avocado.
Preparation Time: 10 minutes
Total Time: 1 hour
Serving Size: 1/2 cup
Ingredients:
2 ripe avocados
1/4 cup unsweetened cocoa powder
1/4 cup maple syrup
1 tsp vanilla extract
Pinch of salt
Directions:
1. Blend avocados, cocoa powder, maple syrup, vanilla extract, and a pinch of salt until smooth.
2. Refrigerate for an hour before serving.
3. Optional: Top with fresh berries or chopped nuts.
Nutritional Info (per serving): Calories: 180 Protein: 3g Carbohydrate: 20g Fat: 12g Sodium: 5mg Potassium: 350mg Fiber: 7g

Pumpkin Spice Energy Bites

A fall-inspired treat with the warmth of pumpkin spice and the energy boost from oats and nuts.
Preparation Time: 15 minutes
Total Time: 1 hour

Serving Size: 2 bites

Ingredients:

1 cup rolled oats (gluten-free)

1/2 cup pumpkin puree

1/4 cup almond butter

2 tbsp maple syrup

1 tsp pumpkin spice

Chopped pecans for rolling (optional)

Directions:

1. Mix oats, pumpkin puree, almond butter, maple syrup, and pumpkin spice.

2. Form into bite-sized balls and roll in chopped pecans if desired.

3. Refrigerate for an hour before serving.

Nutritional Info (per serving): Calories: 160 Protein: 5g Carbohydrate: 18g Fat: 8g Sodium: 15mg Potassium: 180mg Fiber: 4g

Mango Coconut Chia Popsicles

A tropical delight in the form of chia seed popsicles with mango and coconut.

Preparation Time: 15 minutes

 Total Time: 4 hours (freezing time)

 Serving Size: 1 popsicle

Ingredients:

1 cup coconut milk

1/2 cup mango puree

2 tbsp chia seeds

1 tbsp agave syrup

Directions:

1. Mix coconut milk, mango puree, chia seeds, and agave syrup in a bowl.

2. Pour into popsicle molds and freeze for at least 4 hours.

Nutritional Info (per serving): Calories: 80 Protein: 2g Carbohydrate: 10g Fat: 4g Sodium: 10mg Potassium: 90mg Fiber: 2g

Cinnamon Walnut Protein Bars

A flavorful protein bar with the warmth of cinnamon and the crunch of walnuts.

Preparation Time: 20 minutes

Total Time: 2 hours

Serving Size: 1 bar

Ingredients:

1 cup vanilla protein powder
1/2 cup almond flour
1/4 cup chopped walnuts
2 tbsp cinnamon
1/4 cup almond butter
1/4 cup unsweetened applesauce

Directions:

1. Mix protein powder, almond flour, chopped walnuts, and cinnamon in a bowl.
2. Add almond butter and applesauce, combine until a dough forms.
3. Press into a lined pan and refrigerate for 2 hours before cutting into bars.

Nutritional Info (per serving): Calories: 190 Protein: 15g Carbohydrate: 12g Fat: 10g Sodium: 30mg Potassium: 200mg Fiber: 4g

CREAMY CAKE RECIPES

These creamy cakes offer a delicious way to indulge in dessert while staying true to high protein, vegetarian, gluten-free, low sugar, and oil-free requirements. Feel free to make an Adjustments suit your dietary preferences and needs. Enjoy these healthier dessert options!

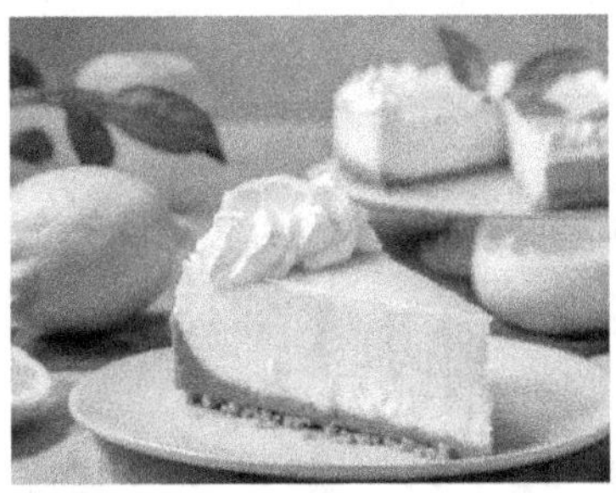

Greek Yogurt Lemon Cheesecake

A tangy and luscious cheesecake with the goodness of Greek yogurt.

Preparation Time: 20 minutes
Cooking Time: 45 minutes
Total Time: 1 hour 5 minutes

Serving Size: 1 slice

Ingredients:

2 cups Greek yogurt

1 cup almond flour (gluten-free)

1/2 cup honey or maple syrup

3 large eggs

Zest and juice of 2 lemons

1 teaspoon vanilla extract

Directions:

1. Preheat the oven to 325°F (163°C) and grease a cake pan.

2. In a bowl, mix Greek yogurt, almond flour, honey, eggs, lemon zest, lemon juice, and vanilla extract.

3. Pour the batter into the pan and bake for about 45 minutes.

4. Allow to cool before slicing.

Nutritional Info (per serving): Calories: 250 Protein: 15g Carbohydrate: 20g Fat: 12g Sodium: 80mg Potassium: 180mg Fiber: 2g

Chocolate Avocado Protein Cake

A rich and moist chocolate cake made with the creamy goodness of avocados.

Preparation Time: 25 minutes

Cooking Time: 30 minutes

Total Time: 55 minutes

Serving Size: 1 slice

Ingredients:

2 ripe avocados, mashed

1 cup almond flour

1/2 cup chocolate protein powder

1/4 cup cocoa powder

1/4 cup honey or agave syrup

3 large eggs

1 teaspoon vanilla extract

Directions:

1. Preheat the oven to 350°F (175°C) and grease a cake pan.

2. In a bowl, combine mashed avocados, almond flour, chocolate protein powder, cocoa powder, honey, eggs, and vanilla extract.

3. Pour into the pan and bake for 30 minutes.

Allow to cool before slicing.

Nutritional Info (per serving): Calories: 280 Protein: 18g Carbohydrate: 20g Fat: 15g Sodium: 40mg Potassium: 320mg Fiber: 6g

Protein-Packed Tofu Vanilla Cake

A light and fluffy vanilla cake made with protein-rich tofu.
Preparation Time: 15 minutes
Cooking Time: 25 minutes
Total Time: 40 minutes
Serving Size: 1 slice
Ingredients:
1 block silken tofu (12 ounces)
1 cup oat flour (gluten-free)
1/2 cup vanilla protein powder
1/4 cup honey or maple syrup
1 teaspoon baking powder
1 teaspoon vanilla extract
Directions:
1. Preheat the oven to 350°F (175°C) and grease a cake pan.
2. Blend silken tofu until smooth.
3. In a bowl, mix blended tofu, oat flour, vanilla protein powder, honey, baking powder, and vanilla extract.
4. Pour into the pan and bake for 25 minutes.
5. Allow to cool before slicing.
Nutritional Info (per serving): Calories: 220 Protein: 20g Carbohydrate: 15g Fat: 10g Sodium: 60mg Potassium: 180mg Fiber: 2g

Coconut Almond Flour Carrot Cake

A moist and nutty carrot cake made with coconut and almond flour.
Preparation Time: 20 minutes
Cooking Time: 40 minutes
Total Time: 1 hour
Serving Size: 1 slice
Ingredients:
2 cups shredded carrots
1 cup almond flour
1/2 cup coconut flour
1/4 cup chopped walnuts
1/4 cup raisins
3 large eggs

1/4 cup honey or agave syrup
1 teaspoon cinnamon
Directions:
1. Preheat the oven to 350°F (175°C) and grease a cake pan.
2. In a bowl, mix shredded carrots, almond flour, coconut flour, chopped walnuts, raisins, eggs, honey, and cinnamon.
3. Pour into the pan and bake for 40 minutes.
4. Remove from the oven and allow to cool before slicing. Enjoy!
Nutritional Info (per serving): Calories: 280 Protein: 15g Carbohydrate: 30g Fat: 12g Sodium: 50mg Potassium: 300mg Fiber: 6g

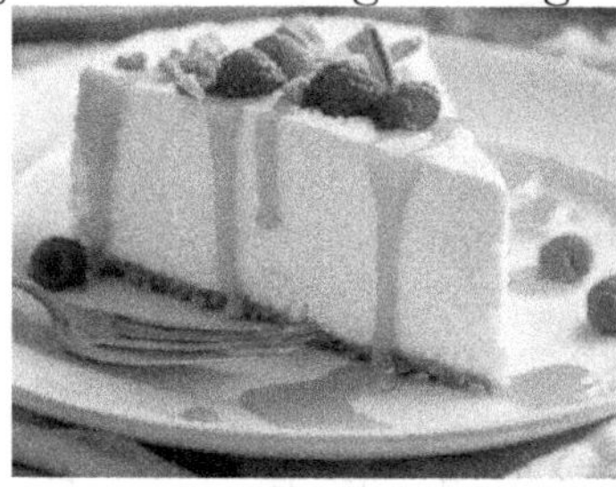

Vanilla Bean Cottage Cheese Cake

A velvety vanilla bean cake with the creaminess of cottage cheese.
Preparation Time: 25 minutes
Cooking Time: 35 minutes
Total Time: 1 hour
Serving Size: 1 slice
Ingredients:
1 1/2 cups low-fat cottage cheese
1 cup almond flour
1/2 cup vanilla protein powder
1/4 cup honey or maple syrup
3 large eggs
1 vanilla bean (seeds scraped)
Directions:
1. Preheat the oven to 325°F (163°C) and grease a cake pan.
2. In a blender, blend cottage cheese until smooth.
3. In a bowl, combine blended cottage cheese, almond flour, vanilla protein powder, honey, eggs, and scraped vanilla bean seeds.
4. Pour into the pan and bake for 35 minutes.
5. Remove from the heat and let it cool before slicing.

*Nutritional Info (per serving): Calories: 250 Protein: 20g Carbohydrate: 18g
Fat: 12g Sodium: 300mg Potassium: 200mg Fiber: 2g*

Peanut Butter Banana Protein Cake

A decadent cake with the classic combination of peanut butter and banana.
Preparation Time: 15 minutes
Cooking Time: 30 minutes
Total Time: 45 minutes
Serving Size: 1 slice
Ingredients:
2 ripe bananas, mashed
1/2 cup peanut butter
1/4 cup almond flour
1/4 cup vanilla protein powder
1/4 cup honey or agave syrup
2 large eggs
1 teaspoon baking powder
Directions:
1/2 teaspoon vanilla extract
Pinch of salt
Directions:
1. Preheat the oven to 350°F (175°C) and grease a cake pan.
2. In a bowl, mix mashed bananas, peanut butter, almond flour,
vanilla protein powder, honey, eggs, baking powder, vanilla extract,
and a pinch of salt.
3. Pour into the pan and bake for 30 minutes.
4. Remove from the oven and place in a cooling rack to cool before
slicing.
*Nutritional Info (per serving): Calories: 300 Protein: 18g Carbohydrate: 25g
Fat: 16g Sodium: 180mg Potassium: 320mg Fiber: 4g*

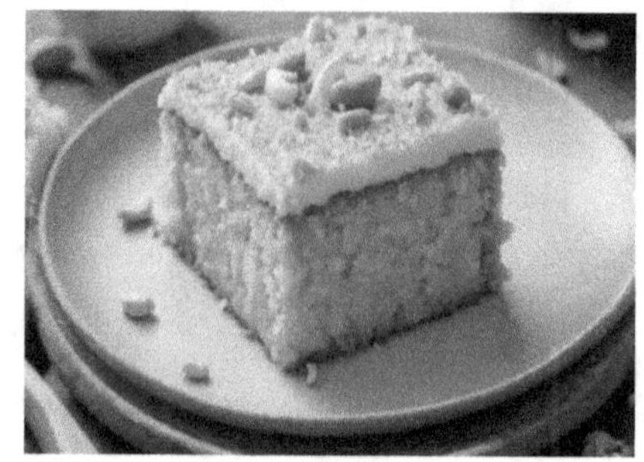

Cashew Coconut Protein Cake

A tropical-inspired cake with the richness of cashews and coconut.
Preparation Time: 20 minutes
Cooking Time: 40 minutes
Total Time: 1 hour
Serving Size: 1 slice
Ingredients:
1 cup cashews, soaked and blended
1/2 cup coconut flour
1/4 cup vanilla protein powder
1/4 cup honey or agave syrup
3 large eggs
1/4 cup shredded coconut
1 teaspoon baking powder
Directions:
1. Preheat the oven to 350°F (175°C) and grease a cake pan.
2. Blend soaked cashews until smooth.
3. In a bowl, mix blended cashews, coconut flour, vanilla protein powder, honey, eggs, shredded coconut, and baking powder.
4. Pour into the pan and bake for 40 minutes.
5. Allow to cool before slicing.
Nutritional Info (per serving): Calories: 280 Protein: 16g Carbohydrate: 25g Fat: 15g Sodium: 90mg Potassium: 300mg Fiber: 5g

Cherry Almond Protein Cake

A delightful cake combining the sweetness of cherries with the nuttiness of almonds.
Preparation Time: 20 minutes
Cooking Time: 35 minutes
Total Time: 55 minutes

Serving Size: 1 slice
Ingredients:
1 cup almond flour
1/2 cup vanilla protein powder
1/4 cup honey or maple syrup
3 large eggs
1/2 cup almond milk
1 teaspoon almond extract
1 cup cherries, fresh or frozen, pitted and halved
Directions:
1. Preheat the oven to 350°F (175°C) and grease a cake pan.
2. In a bowl, mix almond flour, vanilla protein powder, honey, eggs, almond milk, and almond extract.
3. Gently fold in the cherries.
4. Pour the batter into the pan and bake for 35 minutes.
5. Remove the pan from the oven and allow to cool before slicing.
Nutritional Info (per serving): Calories: 260 Protein: 18g Carbohydrate: 22g Fat: 12g Sodium: 50mg Potassium: 230mg Fiber: 4g

Strawberry Shortcake Protein Cake

A healthier twist on classic strawberry shortcake with added protein.
Preparation Time: 15 minutes
Cooking Time: 25 minutes
Total Time: 40 minutes
Serving Size: 1 slice
Ingredients:
1 1/2 cups almond flour
1/2 cup vanilla protein powder
1/4 cup honey or agave syrup
3 large eggs
1/4 cup almond milk
1 teaspoon vanilla extract
1 cup fresh strawberries, sliced
Directions:
1. Preheat the oven to 350°F (175°C) and grease a cake pan.
2. In a bowl, mix almond flour, vanilla protein powder, honey, eggs, almond milk, and vanilla extract.
3. Pour into the pan and bake for 25 minutes.
4. Let it cool in a cooling rack before slicing.

5. Top with sliced strawberries before serving. Enjoy!

Nutritional Info (per serving): Calories: 280 Protein: 20g Carbohydrate: 22g Fat: 14g Sodium: 70mg Potassium: 220mg Fiber: 3g

Blueberry Almond Protein Coffee Cake

A coffee cake filled with juicy blueberries and the crunch of almonds.
Preparation Time: 25 minutes
Cooking Time: 40 minutes
Total Time: 1 hour 5 minutes
Serving Size: 1 slice
Ingredients:
1 1/2 cups almond flour
1/2 cup vanilla protein powder
1/4 cup honey or maple syrup
3 large eggs
1/4 cup almond milk
1 teaspoon almond extract
1 cup fresh or frozen blueberries
1/4 cup sliced almonds
Directions:
1. Preheat the oven to 350°F (175°C) and grease a cake pan.
2. In a bowl, mix almond flour, vanilla protein powder, honey, eggs, almond milk, and almond extract.
3. Gently fold in the blueberries.
4. Pour into the prepared pan, sprinkle sliced almonds on top, and bake for 40 minutes.
5. Remove the cake from the oven and let it cool before slicing.
Nutritional Info (per serving): Calories: 290 Protein: 20g Carbohydrate: 22g Fat: 15g Sodium: 60mg Potassium: 240mg Fiber: 4g

COOKIES RECIPES

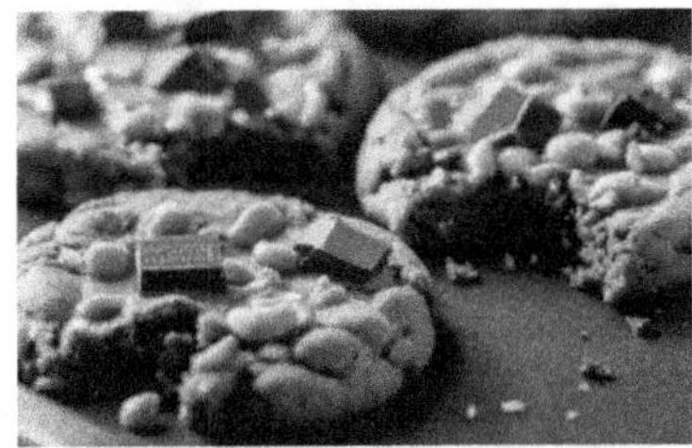

]High Protein Chocolate Peanut Butter Cookies

Indulge in a guilt-free treat with these high-protein, gluten-free, low-sugar, oil-free chocolate peanut butter cookies.

Preparation Time: 15 minutes
Cooking Time: 12 minutes
Total Time: 27 minutes
Serving Size: 2 cookies

Ingredients:

1 cup chickpea flour
1/2 cup chocolate protein powder
1/4 cup unsweetened cocoa powder
1/2 cup natural peanut butter
1/4 cup maple syrup or agave nectar
1/4 cup almond milk
1 teaspoon vanilla extract
1/2 teaspoon baking powder
Pinch of salt
1/4 cup dark chocolate chips (optional)

Directions:

1. Preheat the oven to 350°F (175°C) and properly line a baking sheet with parchment paper.
2. In a bowl, combine chickpea flour, protein powder, cocoa powder, baking powder, and salt.
3. In another bowl, mix peanut butter, maple syrup, almond milk, and vanilla extract until smooth.
4. Combine wet and dry ingredients, folding in chocolate chips if desired.
5. Scoop spoonfuls of dough onto the prepared baking sheet, flattening each with a fork.
6. Bake for 10-12 minutes or until the edges are set.
7. Allow cookies to cool on the sheet for 5 minutes, then transfer to a wire rack to cool completely.

Nutritional Info (per serving): Calories: 180 Protein: 10g (22%) Carbohydrate: 15g (33%) Fat: 9g (45%) Sodium: 120mg Potassium: 180mg Fiber: 3g

Almond Butter Banana Protein Cookies

These Almond Butter Banana Protein Cookies are a delightful blend of sweetness and nuttiness, packed with protein for a satisfying treat.

Preparation Time: 10 minutes

Cooking Time: 15 minutes

Total Time: 25 minutes

Serving Size: 2 cookies

Ingredients:

1 cup almond flour

1/2 cup vanilla protein powder

2 ripe bananas, mashed

1/4 cup almond butter

2 tablespoons maple syrup

1 teaspoon vanilla extract

1/2 teaspoon baking soda

Pinch of salt

1/4 cup chopped almonds (optional)

Directions:

1. Preheat the oven to 350°F (175°C) and properly line a baking sheet with parchment paper.

2. In a bowl, combine almond flour, protein powder, baking soda, and salt.

3. In another bowl, mix mashed bananas, almond butter, maple syrup, and vanilla extract until well combined.

4. Combine wet and dry ingredients, folding in chopped almonds if desired.

5. Drop spoonfuls of dough onto the prepared baking sheet, leaving space between each.

6. Bake for 12-15 minutes or until the edges are golden brown.

7. Allow cookies to cool on the sheet for 5 minutes, then transfer to a wire rack to cool completely.

Nutritional Info (per serving): Calories: 200 Protein: 12g (24%) Carbohydrate: 18g (36%) Fat: 10g (40%) Sodium: 80mg Potassium: 250mg Fiber: 4g

Quinoa Coconut Protein Cookies

These Quinoa Coconut Protein Cookies are a delightful combination of chewy quinoa, coconut, and protein powder, creating a satisfying and nutritious treat.

Preparation Time: 20 minutes
Cooking Time: 15 minutes
Total Time: 35 minutes
Serving Size: 2 cookies
Ingredients:
1 cup cooked quinoa, cooled
1/2 cup vanilla protein powder
1/4 cup coconut flour
1/4 cup shredded coconut
1/4 cup unsweetened applesauce
2 tablespoons maple syrup
1 teaspoon vanilla extract
1/2 teaspoon baking powder
Pinch of salt
1/4 cup chopped walnuts (optional)
Directions:
1. Preheat the oven to 350°F and line a baking sheet with parchment paper.
2. In a bowl, combine cooked quinoa, protein powder, coconut flour, shredded coconut, baking powder, and salt.
3. In another bowl, mix applesauce, maple syrup, and vanilla extract until well combined.
4. Combine wet and dry ingredients, folding in chopped walnuts if desired.
5. Drop spoonfuls of dough onto the prepared baking sheet, shaping them into cookies.
6. Bake for 15 minutes or until the edges are golden brown.
7. Allow cookies to cool on the sheet for 5 minutes, then transfer to a wire rack to cool completely.
Nutritional Info (per serving): Calories: 190 Protein: 11g (23%) Carbohydrate: 20g (42%) Fat: 8g (35%) Sodium: 70mg Potassium: 180mg Fiber: 4g

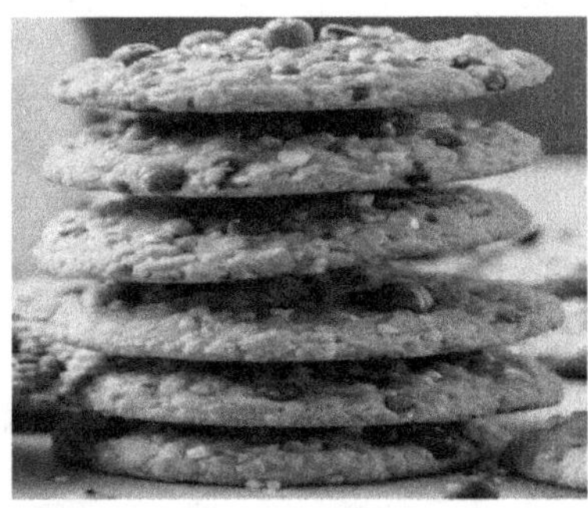

Chia Seed Protein Pudding Cookies

These Chia Seed Protein Pudding Cookies are a nutritious and indulgent treat, combining the goodness of chia seeds and protein powder for a delightful texture.
Preparation Time: 10 minutes
Chilling Time: 1 hour
Total Time: 1 hour 10 minutes
Serving Size: 2 cookies
Ingredients:
1/2 cup chia seeds

1/2 cup vanilla protein powder
1/4 cup unsweetened almond milk
2 tablespoons coconut flour
2 tablespoons maple syrup
1 teaspoon vanilla extract
1/4 cup dark chocolate chips
Pinch of salt
Directions:
1. In a bowl, mix chia seeds, protein powder, coconut flour, and salt.
2. Add almond milk, maple syrup, and vanilla extract to the dry ingredients, stirring until well combined.
3. Allow the mixture to sit for 10 minutes to let the chia seeds absorb the liquid.
4. Fold in dark chocolate chips.
5. Scoop spoonfuls of the mixture onto a parchment-lined tray, shaping them into cookies.
6. Chill in the refrigerator for at least 1 hour to set.
7. Enjoy these protein-packed chia seed cookies!

Nutritional Info (per serving): Calories: 220 Protein: 12g (27%) Carbohydrate: 18g (32%)Fat: 10g (41%) Sodium: 50mg Potassium: 180mg Fiber: 8g

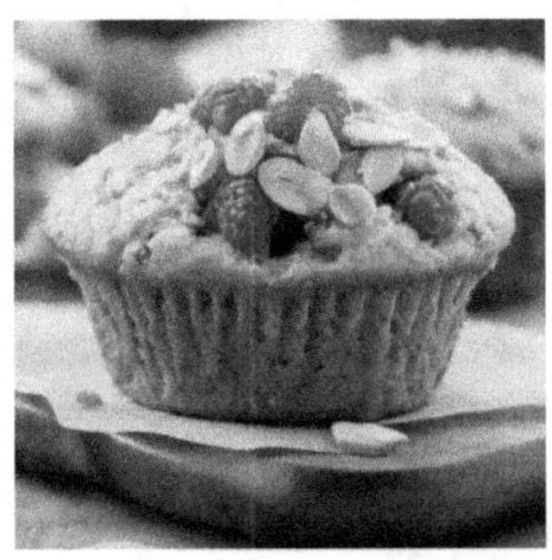

Raspberry Almond Protein Muffin Tops

These Raspberry Almond Protein Muffin Tops are a delightful blend of fruity sweetness and nuttiness, offering a burst of flavor with the goodness of protein and almonds.

Preparation Time: 15 minutes
Baking Time: 18 minutes
Total Time: 33 minutes
Serving Size: 2 muffin tops

Ingredients:

1 cup almond flour
1/2 cup vanilla protein powder
1/4 cup coconut sugar
1 teaspoon baking powder
Pinch of salt
2 tablespoons unsweetened applesauce
1/4 cup almond milk
1 teaspoon almond extract
1/2 cup fresh or frozen raspberries

Directions:

1. Preheat the oven to 350°F (175°C) and line a muffin top pan or baking sheet with parchment paper.
2. In a bowl, combine almond flour, protein powder, coconut sugar, baking powder, and salt.
3. In another bowl, mix applesauce, almond milk, and almond extract until well combined.
4. Combine wet and dry ingredients, folding in raspberries gently.
5. Spoon the batter onto the prepared pan, shaping them into muffin tops.
6. Bake for 18 minutes or until the edges are golden brown.

7. Allow the muffin tops to cool on the pan for 5 minutes, then transfer to a wire rack to cool completely.

Nutritional Info (per serving): Calories: 220 Protein: 14g (31%) Carbohydrate: 16g (29%) Fat: 12g (40%) Sodium: 80mg Potassium: 180mg Fiber: 4g

Peanut Butter Banana Protein Bars

Indulge in the perfect combination of peanut butter and banana with these protein-packed bars. They're an excellent snack for a quick energy boost.

Preparation Time: 15 minutes
Baking Time: 25 minutes
Cooking Time: 1 hour
Total Time: 1 hour 40 minutes
Serving Size: 1 bar

Ingredients:

1 cup gluten-free rolled oats (if necessary)
1/2 cup vanilla protein powder
1/4 cup almond flour
1/4 cup chopped peanuts
1 teaspoon baking powder
Pinch of salt
2 ripe bananas, mashed
1/4 cup natural peanut butter
2 tablespoons maple syrup
1 teaspoon vanilla extract

Directions:

1. Preheat the oven to 350°F (175°C) and line a baking dish with parchment paper.
2. In a bowl, mix rolled oats, protein powder, almond flour, chopped peanuts, baking powder, and salt.
3. In another bowl, combine mashed bananas, peanut butter, maple syrup, and vanilla extract.
4. Combine wet and dry ingredients, stirring until well incorporated.
5. Spread the mixture evenly in the prepared baking dish.
6. Bake for 25 minutes or until the edges are golden brown.
7. Allow the bars to cool in the dish for 10 minutes, then transfer to a wire rack to cool completely.
8. Once cooled, cut into bars. Serve and enjoy!

Nutritional Info (per serving): Calories: 180 Protein: 10g (22%) Carbohydrate: 20g (44%) Fat: 8g (34%) Sodium: 90mg Potassium: 220mg Fiber: 3g

Vanilla Cinnamon Chia Seed Protein Bites

Satisfy your sweet cravings with these Vanilla Cinnamon Chia Seed Protein Bites. Packed with protein and healthy fats, they make for a perfect energy-boosting snack.

Preparation Time: 15 minutes
Chilling Time: 30 minutes
Total Time: 45 minutes
Serving Size: 2 bites
Ingredients:
1/2 cup chia seeds
1/2 cup vanilla protein powder
1/4 cup unsweetened almond butter
2 tablespoons maple syrup
1 teaspoon vanilla extract
1/2 teaspoon ground cinnamon
Pinch of salt
Shredded coconut for rolling (optional)
Directions:
1. In a bowl, mix chia seeds, protein powder, cinnamon, and salt.
2. In a separate microwave-safe bowl, warm almond butter for about 20 seconds until softened.
3. Add almond butter, maple syrup, and vanilla extract to the dry ingredients, stirring until well combined.
4. Allow the mixture to sit for 5 minutes to let the chia seeds absorb the liquid.
5. Roll the mixture into bite-sized balls and, if desired, roll them in shredded coconut.
6. Place the bites on a plate and chill in the refrigerator for at least 30 minutes to set.
7. Enjoy these vanilla-infused, cinnamon-spiced protein bites!
Nutritional Info (per serving): Calories: 160 Protein: 10g (25%) Carbohydrate: 12g (30%) Fat: 8g (45%) Sodium: 50mg Potassium: 120mg Fiber: 6g

Matcha Protein Energy Balls

Elevate your snack game with these Matcha Protein Energy Balls. Packed with the antioxidant goodness of matcha and protein, they make for a perfect on-the-go treat.

Preparation Time: 15 minutes
Chilling Time: 30 minutes
Total Time: 45 minutes
Serving Size: 2 energy balls
Ingredients:

1/2 cup rolled oats (certified gluten-free, if necessary)
1/2 cup vanilla protein powder
2 tablespoons almond flour
1 tablespoon matcha powder
1/4 cup almond butter
2 tablespoons maple syrup
1 teaspoon vanilla extract
Pinch of salt
Crushed pistachios for coating (optional)
Directions:
1. In a food processor, combine rolled oats, protein powder, almond flour, matcha powder, and salt. Pulse until well combined.
2. Add almond butter, maple syrup, and vanilla extract to the dry mixture. Pulse until a dough-like consistency forms.
3. Scoop out spoonfuls of the mixture and roll them into bite-sized balls.
4. If desired, roll each ball in crushed pistachios for added texture.
5. Place the energy balls on a plate and chill in the refrigerator for at least 30 minutes to firm up.
6. Enjoy these vibrant and energizing matcha protein treats!
Nutritional Info (per serving): Calories: 160 Protein: 10g (25%) Carbohydrate: 14g (35%) Fat: 8g (40%) Sodium: 60mg Potassium: 130mg Fiber: 3g

Blueberry Protein Muffins

Enjoy the antioxidant-rich goodness of blueberries in these protein-packed muffins. They're perfect for a quick and satisfying breakfast or snack.
Preparation Time: 15 minutes
Baking Time: 20 minutes
Total Time: 35 minutes
Serving Size: 1 muffin
Ingredients:
1 cup almond flour
1/2 cup vanilla protein powder
1/4 cup coconut sugar
1 teaspoon baking powder
Pinch of salt
2 ripe bananas, mashed
1/4 cup unsweetened applesauce

1 teaspoon vanilla extract
1/2 cup fresh blueberries
Directions:
1. Preheat the oven to 350°F (175°C) and properly line a muffin tin with paper towel.
2. In a bowl, mix almond flour, protein powder, coconut sugar, baking powder, and salt.
3. In another bowl, combine mashed bananas, applesauce, and vanilla extract.
4. Combine wet and dry ingredients, stirring until well incorporated.
5. Gently fold in fresh blueberries.
6. Spoon the batter into the muffin cups, filling each about two-thirds full.
7. Bake for 18-20 minutes or until a toothpick inserted into the center comes out clean.
8. Allow the muffins to cool in the tin for 5 minutes, then transfer to a wire rack to cool completely.
Nutritional Info (per serving): Calories: 180 Protein: 12g (27%) Carbohydrate: 18g (36%) Fat: 8g (37%) Sodium: 90mg Potassium: 220mg Fiber: 4g

Chocolate Avocado Protein Pudding

Indulge in a creamy and decadent Chocolate Avocado Protein Pudding. Packed with healthy fats and protein, this dessert is a guilt-free delight.
Preparation Time: 10 minutes
Chilling Time: 2 hours
Total Time: 2 hours 10 minutes
Serving Size: 1/2 cup
Ingredients:
2 ripe avocados
1/4 cup cocoa powder (unsweetened)
1/4 cup chocolate protein powder
1/4 cup maple syrup or agave nectar
1 teaspoon vanilla extract
Pinch of salt
1/4 cup almond milk (or any plant-based milk)
Directions:
1. In a food processor, blend avocados until smooth.

2. Add cocoa powder, protein powder, maple syrup, vanilla extract, and a pinch of salt to the avocados. Blend until well combined.
3. While blending, gradually add almond milk until the mixture reaches a creamy and pudding-like consistency.
4. Taste and adjust sweetness if needed by adding more maple syrup.
5. Transfer the pudding to serving cups and refrigerate for at least 2 hours to chill and set.
6. Serve chilled, optionally topped with fresh berries or a sprinkle of chopped nuts.

Nutritional Info (per serving): Calories: 220 Protein: 10g (18%) Carbohydrate: 20g (36%) Fat: 15g (46%) Sodium: 50mg Potassium: 540mg Fiber: 8g

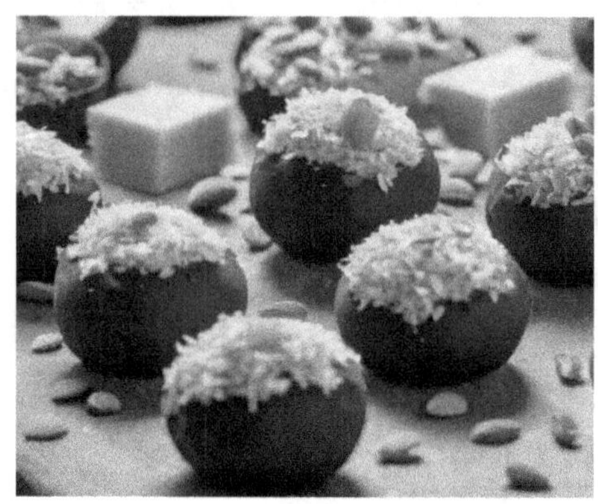

Coconut Almond Protein Truffles

Indulge in these Coconut Almond Protein Truffles for a burst of nutty goodness and protein-packed satisfaction. These no-bake truffles are perfect for a guilt-free treat.

Preparation Time: 15 minutes
Chilling Time: 1 hour
Total Time: 1 hour 15 minutes
Serving Size: 2 truffles

Ingredients:

1/2 cup almond flour
1/2 cup vanilla protein powder
1/4 cup shredded coconut (plus extra for rolling)
2 tablespoons almond butter
2 tablespoons maple syrup
1 teaspoon vanilla extract
Pinch of salt

Directions:

1. In a bowl, combine almond flour, protein powder, shredded coconut, and a pinch of salt.
2. Add almond butter, maple syrup, and vanilla extract to the dry mixture. Stir until a dough-like consistency forms.
3. Take small portions of the mixture and roll them into bite-sized truffles.
4. Roll each truffle in shredded coconut for a coating.
5. Place the truffles on a plate and chill in the refrigerator for at least 1 hour to set.

6. Enjoy these delightful Coconut Almond Protein Truffles as a snack or dessert.

Nutritional Info (per serving): Calories: 180 Protein: 12g (27%) Carbohydrate: 14g (31%) Fat: 10g (42%) Sodium: 60mg Potassium: 130mg Fiber: 3g

Pumpkin Spice Protein Bars

Embrace the flavors of fall with these Pumpkin Spice Protein Bars. Packed with protein and the warmth of spices, these bars make for a satisfying and seasonal treat.

Preparation Time: 15 minutes
Baking Time: 25 minutes
Cooking Time: 1 hour
Total Time: 1 hour 40 minutes
Serving Size: 1 bar

Ingredients:

1 cup pumpkin puree (canned or homemade)
1/2 cup vanilla protein powder
1/4 cup almond flour
1/4 cup coconut flour
1/4 cup maple syrup
2 tablespoons unsweetened applesauce
1 teaspoon pumpkin pie spice
1/2 teaspoon baking soda
Pinch of salt
Chopped pecans for topping (optional)

Directions:

1. Preheat the oven to 350°F (175°C) and line a baking pan with parchment paper.
2. In a bowl, mix pumpkin puree, protein powder, almond flour, coconut flour, pumpkin pie spice, baking soda, and salt.
3. Add maple syrup and applesauce to the dry mixture, stirring until well combined.
4. Properly spread the batter evenly in the prepared baking pan.
5. If desired, sprinkle chopped pecans on top for added crunch.
6. Bake for 25 minutes or until a toothpick inserted into the center comes out clean.
7. Allow the bars to cool in the dish for 10 minutes, then transfer to a wire rack to cool completely.
8. Once cooled, cut into bars and enjoy the fall flavors!

Nutritional Info (per serving): Calories: 190 Protein: 12g (25%) Carbohydrate: 18g (33%) Fat: 8g (42%) Sodium: 120mg Potassium: 180mg Fiber: 4g

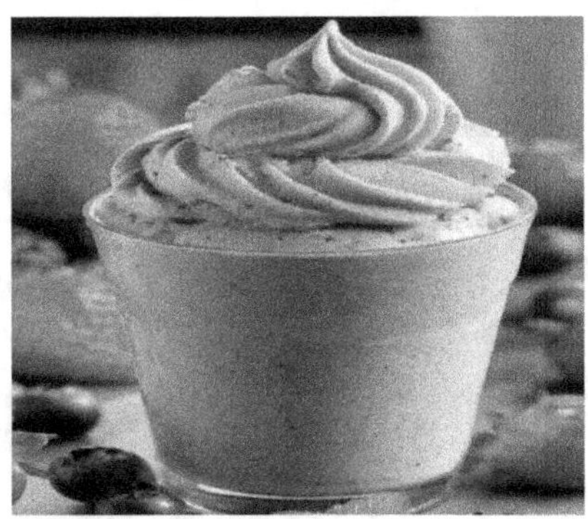

Berry Protein Nice Cream

Cool down with this refreshing and protein-packed Berry Nice Cream. A guilt-free frozen treat that's perfect for satisfying your sweet tooth.

Preparation Time: 10 minutes

Freezing Time: 4 hours

Total Time: 4 hours 10 minutes

Serving Size: 1 cup

Ingredients:

1 cup mixed berries (strawberries, blueberries, raspberries)

1/2 cup vanilla protein powder

1 ripe banana, sliced and frozen

1/4 cup unsweetened almond milk

1 teaspoon lemon juice

1 tablespoon chia seeds (optional)

Directions:

1. In a blender, combine mixed berries, frozen banana slices, vanilla protein powder, almond milk, and lemon juice.

2. Blend until smooth and creamy. Stop and check if the mixture is too thick and add a little more almond milk.

3. If using, stir in chia seeds for added texture.

4. Pour the nice cream into a shallow dish or ice cream container.

5. Freeze for at least 4 hours or until set.

6. Allow the nice cream to thaw for a few minutes before scooping and serving.

7. Garnish with fresh berries or a sprinkle of chia seeds, if desired.

Nutritional Info (per serving): Calories: 220 Protein: 18g (32%) Carbohydrate: 25g (45%) Fat: 7g (23%) Sodium: 90mg Potassium: 450mg Fiber: 7g

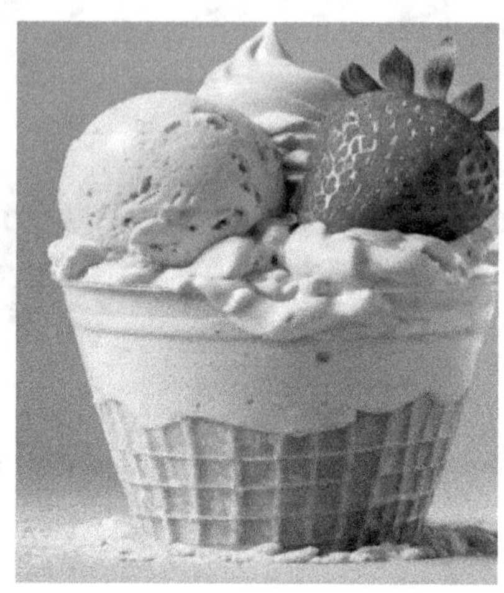

Strawberry Protein Nice Cream

Indulge in the creamy goodness of Strawberry Protein Nice Cream, a guilt-free frozen treat bursting with fruity flavors.
Preparation Time: 10 minutes
Total Time: 4 hours (freezing time included)
Serving Size: 1 cup
Ingredients:
2 cups frozen strawberries
1/2 cup vanilla protein powder
1/4 cup unsweetened almond milk
1 tablespoon maple syrup (optional)
Directions:
1. In a blender, combine frozen strawberries, vanilla protein powder, and almond milk.
2. Blend until smooth, adding more almond milk if necessary.
3. Optionally, add maple syrup for sweetness and blend again.
4. Transfer the mixture into a freezer-safe container and freeze for at least 4 hours.
5. Scoop into a bowl and enjoy this luscious Strawberry Protein Nice Cream!
Nutritional Info (per serving - 1 cup): Calories: 150 Protein: 15g (40%) Carbohydrate: 20g (48%) Fat: 1g (12%) Sodium: 20mg Potassium: 320mg Fiber: 5g

Mango Protein Popsicles

Beat the heat with Mango Protein Popsicles, a tropical delight that combines the sweetness of mango with a protein boost.
Preparation Time: 15 minutes
Freezing Time: 4 hours

Total Time: 4 hours 15 minutes
Serving Size: 1 popsicle
Ingredients:
1 cup fresh or frozen mango chunks
1/2 cup vanilla protein powder
1/2 cup coconut water
1 tablespoon lime juice
Zest of 1 lime (optional)
Directions:
1. In a blender, combine mango chunks, vanilla protein powder, coconut water, lime juice, and lime zest.
Blend until smooth.
2. Pour the mixture into popsicle molds and freeze for at least 4 hours.
3. Run molds under warm water to release the popsicles.
4. Savor the refreshing taste of Mango Protein Popsicles!
Nutritional Info (per serving - 1 Popsicle): Calories: 90 Protein: 10g (44%) Carbohydrate: 12g (48%) Fat: 1g (8%) Sodium: 30mg Potassium: 230mg Fiber: 2g

Blueberry Protein Parfait

Layered with the goodness of blueberries, yogurt, and protein, the Blueberry Protein Parfait is a delightful and nutritious treat.
Preparation Time: 10 minutes
Total Time: 10 minutes
Serving Size: 1 parfait
Ingredients:
1 cup dairy-free yogurt
1/2 cup blueberries (fresh or frozen)
1/4 cup granola (gluten-free)
1/4 cup vanilla protein powder
1 tablespoon almond butter (optional)
Directions:
1. In a glass, layer half of the yogurt.
2. Add half of the blueberries and sprinkle with granola.
3. Mix vanilla protein powder with the remaining yogurt and layer it on top.

4. Finish with the rest of the blueberries and a drizzle of almond butter if desired.
5. Repeat for additional servings.
6. Enjoy this delicious and protein-packed Blueberry Protein Parfait!

Nutritional Info (per serving - 1 parfait): Calories: 300 Protein: 20g (32%) Carbohydrate: 35g (40%) Fat: 10g (28%) Sodium: 120mg Potassium: 320mg Fiber: 6g

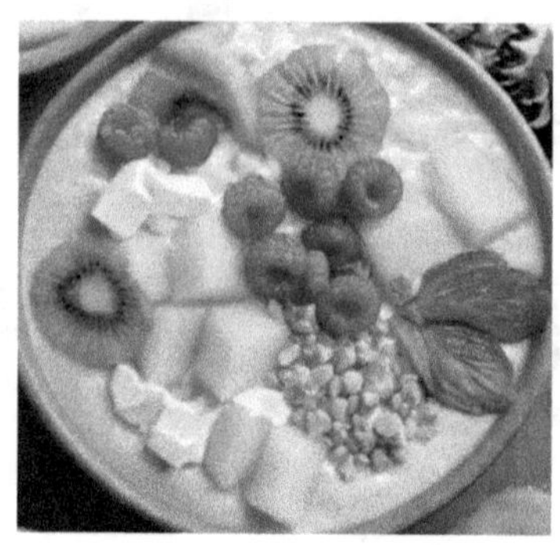

Pineapple Protein Smoothie Bowl

Start your day with a tropical twist! This Pineapple Protein Smoothie Bowl is a refreshing and protein-packed way to fuel your morning.

Preparation Time: 10 minutes

Total Time: 10 minutes

Serving Size: 1 bowl

Ingredients:

1 cup frozen pineapple chunks

1/2 cup vanilla protein powder

1/2 cup coconut milk

1 ripe banana

Toppings: sliced kiwi, shredded coconut, chia seeds

Directions:

1. In a blender, combine frozen pineapple chunks, vanilla protein powder, coconut milk, and ripe banana.

2. Blend until smooth and creamy.

3. Pour the smoothie into a bowl.

Top with sliced kiwi, shredded coconut, and chia seeds.

Enjoy this tropical and protein-rich Pineapple Protein Smoothie Bowl.

Nutritional Info (per serving): Calories: 280 Protein: 25g (36%) Carbohydrate: 30g (40%) Fat: 8g (24%) Sodium: 50mg Potassium: 520mg Fiber: 5g

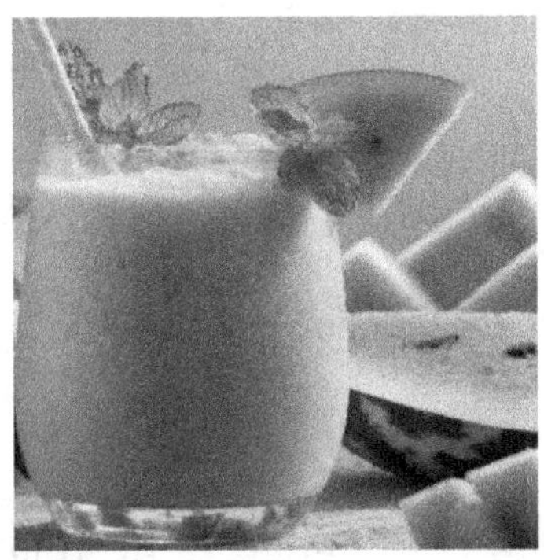

Watermelon Mint Protein Slushie

Cool off with a refreshing Watermelon Mint Protein Slushie. This hydrating treat is perfect for hot days and offers a protein boost.

Preparation Time: 5 minutes

Total Time: 5 minutes

Serving Size: 1 slushie

Ingredients:

2 cups cubed seedless watermelon

1/2 cup vanilla protein powder

1 tablespoon fresh mint leaves

Ice cubes

Directions:

1. In a blender, combine cubed watermelon, vanilla protein powder, fresh mint leaves, and ice cubes.

2. Blend until smooth and slushie-like.

3. Pour into a glass and garnish with a mint sprig if desired.

4. Enjoy this hydrating and protein-packed Watermelon Mint Protein Slushie.

Nutritional Info (per serving): Calories: 180 Protein: 20g (44%) Carbohydrate: 20g (36%) Fat: 1g (20%) Sodium: 30mg Potassium: 450mg Fiber: 1g

Cherry Chocolate Protein Chia Pudding

Indulge in the decadence of Cherry Chocolate Protein Chia Pudding, a delightful combination of flavors and textures.

Preparation Time: 10 minutes (+ chilling time)

Total Time: 4 hours

Serving Size: 1/2 cup

Ingredients:

1/4 cup chia seeds

1 cup almond milk
1/4 cup chocolate protein powder
1/2 cup pitted cherries, chopped
1 tablespoon cacao nibs (optional)
Directions:
1. In a bowl, whisk together chia seeds, almond milk, and chocolate protein powder.
2. Let the mixture sit for 10 minutes, stirring occasionally.
3. Fold in chopped cherries and cacao nibs.
4. Refrigerate for at least 4 hours or overnight until it reaches a pudding-like consistency.
5. Serve in a bowl or jar and enjoy this Cherry Chocolate Protein Chia Pudding.
Nutritional Info (per serving - 1/2 cup): Calories: 220 Protein: 15g (27%) Carbohydrate: 25g (45%) Fat: 8g (28%) Sodium: 30mg Potassium: 220mg Fiber: 9g

Banana Berry Protein Muffins

These Banana Berry Protein Muffins are a delightful blend of ripe bananas and juicy berries, packed with protein for a satisfying treat.
Preparation Time: 15 minutes
Baking Time: 20 minutes
Total Time: 35 minutes
Serving Size: 1 muffin
Ingredients:
2 ripe bananas, mashed
1/4 cup vanilla protein powder
1 cup gluten-free oat flour
1/2 cup mixed berries (blueberries, raspberries, strawberries)
1/4 cup almond milk
1 teaspoon baking powder
1/2 teaspoon cinnamon
Pinch of salt
Directions:
1. Preheat the oven to 350°F (175°C) and line a muffin tin with liners.
2. In a bowl, combine mashed bananas, vanilla protein powder, oat flour, almond milk, baking powder, cinnamon, and a pinch of salt.
3. Gently fold in mixed berries.

4. Spoon the batter into muffin cups.
5. Bake for 20 minutes or until a toothpick comes out clean.
6. Allow to cool before enjoying these Banana Berry Protein Muffins!
Nutritional Info (per serving - 1 muffin): Calories: 120 Protein: 8g (27%) Carbohydrate: 20g (53%) Fat: 2g (20%) Sodium: 50mg Potassium: 160mg Fiber: 3g

Apple Cinnamon Protein Energy Bites

Experience the warmth of apple and cinnamon in these protein-packed energy bites, perfect for a quick and wholesome snack.

Preparation Time: 15 minutes

Total Time: 1 hour (chilling time included)

Serving Size: 2 bites

Ingredients:

1 cup diced apples

1/4 cup vanilla protein powder

1/2 cup gluten-free rolled oats

2 tablespoons almond butter

1 tablespoon maple syrup

1 teaspoon ground cinnamon

Pinch of nutmeg

Directions:

1. In a food processor, combine diced apples, vanilla protein powder, rolled oats, almond butter, maple syrup, ground cinnamon, and a pinch of nutmeg.

2. Pulse until the mixture forms a dough-like consistency.

3. Roll the mixture into bite-sized balls and place on a tray.

4. Refrigerate for at least 1 hour to set.

5. Enjoy these Apple Cinnamon Protein Energy Bites as a nutritious snack!

Nutritional Info (per serving - 2 bites): Calories: 150 Protein: 10g (27%) Carbohydrate: 20g (50%) Fat: 6g (36%) Sodium: 20mg Potassium: 120mg Fiber: 4g

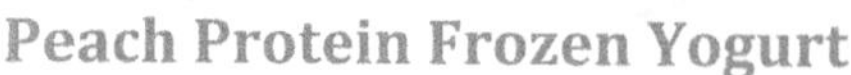

Peach Protein Frozen Yogurt

Cool down with the sweet and creamy goodness of Peach Protein Frozen Yogurt, a satisfying dessert with a protein kick.

Preparation Time: 10 minutes

Freezing Time: 4 hours
Total Time: 4 hours 10 minutes
Serving Size: 1/2 cup
Ingredients:
1 cup frozen peach slices
1/2 cup plain Greek yogurt
1/4 cup vanilla protein powder
1 tablespoon honey (optional)
Directions:
1. In a blender, combine frozen peach slices, Greek yogurt, vanilla protein powder, and honey (if using).
2. Blend until smooth and creamy.
3. Transfer the mixture into a freezer-safe container and freeze for at least 4 hours.
4. Scoop into a bowl and enjoy this Peach Protein Frozen Yogurt!
Nutritional Info (per serving - 1/2 cup): Calories: 160 Protein: 15g (37%) Carbohydrate: 20g (48%) Fat: 2g (15%) Sodium: 30mg Potassium: 220mg Fiber: 2g

Avocado Chocolate Protein Pudding

Indulge in a rich and creamy Avocado Chocolate Protein Pudding that combines the goodness of avocado with the decadence of chocolate.
Preparation Time: 10 minutes
Chilling Time: 1 hour
Total Time: 1 hour 10 minutes
Serving Size: 1/2 cup
Ingredients:
1 ripe avocado
1/4 cup chocolate protein powder
2 tablespoons unsweetened cocoa powder
2 tablespoons maple syrup
1/2 teaspoon vanilla extract
Pinch of sea salt
Fresh berries for topping
Directions:

1. In a food processor, blend the ripe avocado until smooth.
2. Add chocolate protein powder, cocoa powder, maple syrup, vanilla extract, and a pinch of sea salt.

3. Blend until well combined and creamy.
4. Transfer the pudding into serving bowls and refrigerate for at least 1 hour.
5. Top with fresh berries before serving.
6. Enjoy this decadent and protein-rich Avocado Chocolate Protein Pudding!

Nutritional Info (per serving - 1/2 cup): Calories: 220 Protein: 15g (27%) Carbohydrate: 20g (45%) Fat: 12g (42%) Sodium: 20mg Potassium: 490mg Fiber: 7g

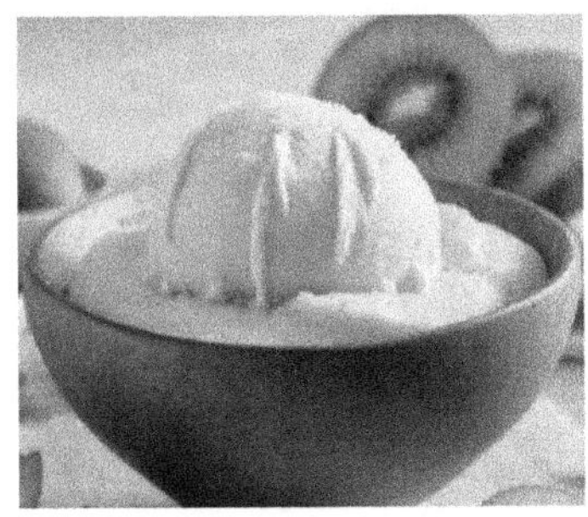

Kiwi Protein Sorbet

Savor the refreshing taste of Kiwi Protein Sorbet, a delightful frozen treat bursting with the goodness of kiwi and protein.

Preparation Time: 15 minutes
Freezing Time: 4 hours
Total Time: 4 hours 15 minutes
Serving Size: 1/2 cup

Ingredients:

2 cups peeled and sliced kiwi
1/4 cup vanilla protein powder
2 tablespoons agave syrup or honey
1 tablespoon lime juice
Fresh mint leaves for garnish

Directions:

1. In a blender, combine sliced kiwi, vanilla protein powder, agave syrup or honey, and lime juice.
Blend until smooth.
2. Pour the mixture into a freezer-safe container and freeze for about 4 hours or more.
3. Use a fork to scrape and fluff the sorbet before serving.
4. Garnish with fresh mint leaves.
5. Enjoy this zesty and protein-packed Kiwi Protein Sorbet!

Nutritional Info (per serving - 1/2 cup): Calories: 120 Protein: 8g (30%) Carbohydrate: 25g (58%) Fat: 1g (12%) Sodium: 10mg Potassium: 410mg Fiber: 4g

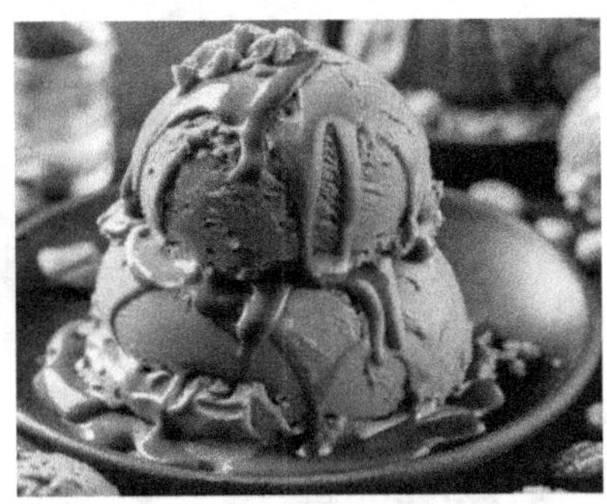

Chocolate Peanut Butter Protein Ice Cream

Indulge in the richness of chocolate and the creaminess of peanut butter with this protein-packed ice cream.

Preparation Time: 10 minutes
Freezing Time: 4 hours
Total Time: 4 hours 10 minutes
Serving Size: 1 cup

Ingredients:
2 ripe bananas, sliced and frozen
1/4 cup chocolate protein powder
2 tablespoons natural peanut butter
1/4 cup almond milk

Directions:
1. In a blender, combine frozen banana slices, chocolate protein powder, peanut butter, and almond milk.
2. Blend until smooth and creamy.
3. Transfer the mixture into a freezer-safe container and freeze for at least 4 hours.
4. Allow the ice cream to thaw for a few minutes before serving.
Nutritional Info (per serving): Calories: 250 Protein: 18g (29%) Carbohydrate: 35g (50%) Fat: 8g (29%) Sodium: 80mg Potassium: 600mg Fiber: 5g

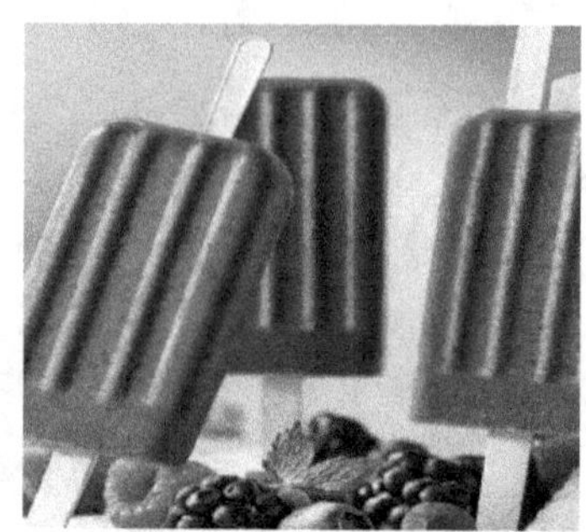

Mixed Berry Protein Popsicles

Beat the heat with these refreshing and fruity mixed berry protein popsicles.

Preparation Time: 15 minutes

Freezing Time: 3 hours

Total Time: 3 hours 15 minutes

Serving Size: 1 popsicle

Ingredients:

1 cup mixed berries (strawberries, blueberries, raspberries)

1/2 cup vanilla protein powder

1 cup unsweetened almond milk

1 tablespoon maple syrup (optional)

Directions:

1. In a blender, combine mixed berries, vanilla protein powder, almond milk, and maple syrup.

Blend the mixture until smooth.

2. Pour the mixture into popsicle molds and freeze for at least 3 hours.

3. Run molds under warm water to release the popsicles.

Nutritional Info (per serving): Calories: 120 Protein: 12g (40%) Carbohydrate: 15g (50%) Fat: 2g (10%) Sodium: 90mg Potassium: 250mg Fiber: 4g

Mango Coconut Protein Sorbet

Transport yourself to a tropical paradise with this luscious mango and coconut protein sorbet.

Preparation Time: 15 minutes

Freezing Time: 5 hours

Total Time: 5 hours 15 minutes

Serving Size: 1/2 cup

Ingredients:
2 cups frozen mango chunks
1/4 cup vanilla protein powder
1/2 cup coconut water
1 tablespoon shredded coconut
Directions:
1. In a blender, combine frozen mango chunks, vanilla protein powder, and coconut water and blend until smooth.
2. Transfer the mixture into a freezer-safe container, sprinkle with shredded coconut, and freeze for at least 5 hours.
3. Allow the sorbet to thaw for a few minutes before serving.
Nutritional Info (per serving): Calories: 160 Protein: 10g (25%) Carbohydrate: 25g (55%) Fat: 2g (10%) Sodium: 40mg Potassium: 450mg Fiber: 4g

Vanilla Almond Protein Nice Cream Bars

Delight in the classic combination of vanilla and almond with these creamy and protein-packed nice cream bars.
Preparation Time: 15 minutes
Freezing Time: 4 hours
Total Time: 4 hours 15 minutes
Serving Size: 1 bar
Ingredients:
2 ripe bananas, sliced and frozen
1/2 cup vanilla protein powder
1/4 cup almond flour
1/4 cup almond butter
1/4 cup unsweetened almond milk
Directions:
1. In a blender, combine frozen banana slices, vanilla protein powder, almond flour, almond butter, and almond milk and blend until smooth.
2. Pour the mixture into a rectangular mold or tray, spreading it evenly.
3. Freeze for at least 4 hours.
4. Slice into bars and enjoy this guilt-free frozen treat.
Nutritional Info (per serving): Calories: 220 Protein: 15g (27%) Carbohydrate: 20g (36%) Fat: 9g (37%) Sodium: 70mg Potassium: 450mg Fiber: 5g

Chia Seed Protein Berry Popsicles

These chia seed-infused popsicles offer a refreshing burst of mixed berries and the added benefit of protein.

Preparation Time: 20 minutes
Freezing Time: 4 hours
Total Time: 4 hours 20 minutes
Serving Size: 1 popsicle

Ingredients:

1 cup mixed berries (strawberries, blueberries, raspberries)
1/2 cup vanilla protein powder
2 tablespoons chia seeds
1 cup unsweetened coconut water

Directions:

1. In a blender, combine mixed berries, vanilla protein powder, chia seeds, and coconut water.
2. Blend the mixture until smooth.
3. Pour the mixture into popsicle molds and freeze for at least 4 hours.
4. Run molds under warm water to release the popsicles.

Nutritional Info (per serving): Calories: 150 Protein: 12g (32%) Carbohydrate: 18g (48%) Fat: 4g (20%) Sodium: 30mg Potassium: 300mg Fiber: 6g

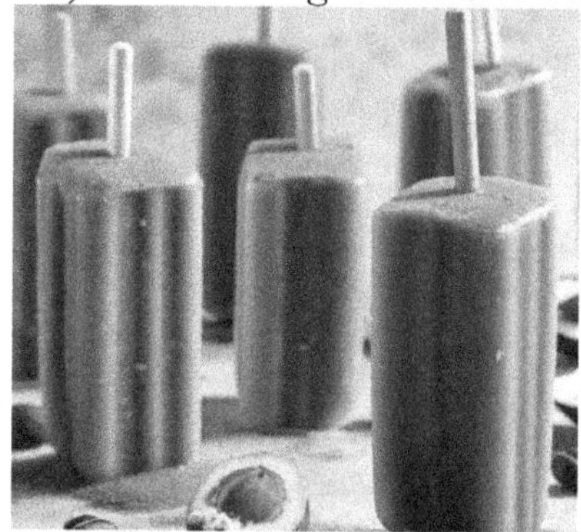

Coffee Hazelnut Protein Ice Pops

Satisfy your coffee cravings with these refreshing and protein-rich coffee hazelnut ice pops.

Preparation Time: 10 minutes
Freezing Time: 4 hours
Total Time: 4 hours 10 minutes
Serving Size: 1 ice pop

Ingredients:
1 cup brewed and chilled coffee
1/2 cup vanilla protein powder
2 tablespoons hazelnut butter
1 tablespoon maple syrup (optional)
Directions:
1. In a bowl, mix chilled coffee, vanilla protein powder, hazelnut butter, and maple syrup.
2. Stir until the mixture is well combined.
3. Pour the mixture into ice pop molds and freeze for at least 4 hours.
4. Run molds under warm water to release the ice pops. Enjoy!
Nutritional Info (per serving): Calories: 120 Protein: 10g (33%) Carbohydrate: 8g (27%) Fat: 5g (40%) Sodium: 20mg Potassium: 220mg Fiber: 2g

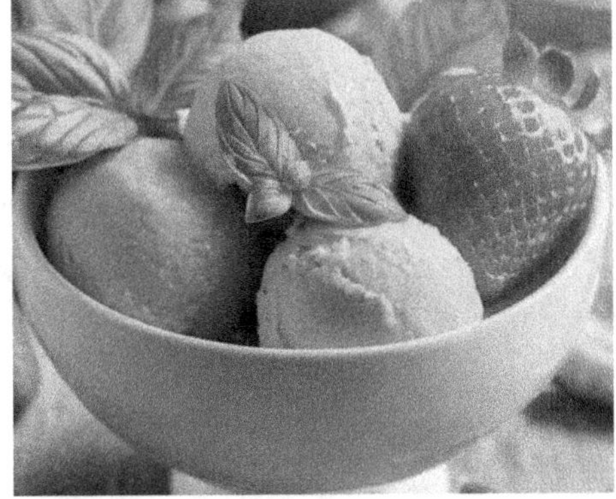

Strawberry Basil Protein Sorbet

Experience a unique blend of sweet and savory with this refreshing Strawberry Basil Protein Sorbet, offering a delightful twist on traditional flavors.
Preparation Time: 15 minutes
Freezing Time: 5 hours
Total Time: 5 hours 15 minutes
Serving Size: 1/2 cup
Ingredients:
2 cups fresh strawberries, hulled
1/2 cup vanilla protein powder
1/4 cup fresh basil leaves
1/4 cup coconut water
1 tablespoon lemon juice

1 tablespoon agave nectar (optional)

Directions:

1. In a blender, combine fresh strawberries, vanilla protein powder, basil leaves, coconut water, lemon juice, and agave nectar.
2. Blend the mixture until smooth.
3. Transfer the mixture into a freezer-safe container and freeze for at least 5 hours.
4. Allow the sorbet to thaw for a few minutes before serving.

Nutritional Info (per serving): Calories: 140 Protein: 10g (28%) Carbohydrate: 20g (50%) Fat: 2g (14%) Sodium: 40mg Potassium: 300mg Fiber: 4g

Mint Chocolate Chip Protein Nice Cream

Indulge in the classic combination of mint and chocolate with this protein-packed nice cream, offering a healthier twist on a favorite flavor.
Preparation Time: 15 minutes
Freezing Time: 4 hours
Total Time: 4 hours 15 minutes
Serving Size: 1 cup
Ingredients:
2 ripe bananas, sliced and frozen
1/2 cup vanilla protein powder
1/2 teaspoon peppermint extract
2 tablespoons dark chocolate chips (sugar-free)
Directions:
1. In a blender, combine frozen banana slices, vanilla protein powder, and peppermint extract.
2. Blend until smooth.
4. 3. Stir in dark chocolate chips.
3. Transfer the mixture into a freezer-safe container and freeze for at least 4 hours.
Allow the nice cream to thaw for a few minutes before serving.
Nutritional Info (per serving): Calories: 230 Protein: 15g (26%) Carbohydrate: 35g (57%) Fat: 6g (17%) Sodium: 50mgPotassium: 500mg Fiber: 5g

Pineapple Coconut Protein Popsicles

Transport yourself to a tropical paradise with these exotic Pineapple Coconut Protein Popsicles, providing a refreshing burst of flavor.
Preparation Time: 15 minutes
Freezing Time: 4 hours
Total Time: 4 hours 15 minutes
Serving Size: 1 popsicle
Ingredients:
1 cup fresh pineapple chunks
1/2 cup vanilla protein powder
1/2 cup coconut milk
1 tablespoon shredded coconut (unsweetened)
Directions:
1. In a blender, combine fresh pineapple chunks, vanilla protein powder, and coconut milk.

2. Blend until smooth.

3. Pour the mixture into popsicle molds and sprinkle shredded coconut on top.

4. Freeze for at least 4 hours.

5. Run molds under warm water to release the popsicles.

Nutritional Info (per serving): Calories: 180 Protein: 14g (31%) Carbohydrate: 20g (44%) Fat: 7g (25%) Sodium: 20mg Potassium: 350mg Fiber: 3g

Raspberry Lemon Protein Sorbet

Indulge in the zesty combination of raspberries and lemon with this protein-packed sorbet, offering a burst of fruity freshness.

Preparation Time: 15 minutes

Freezing Time: 5 hours

Total Time: 5 hours 15 minutes

Serving Size: 1/2 cup

Ingredients:

2 cups fresh or frozen raspberries

1/2 cup vanilla protein powder

Zest and juice of 1 lemon

1/4 cup coconut water

2 tablespoons agave nectar (optional)

Directions:

1. In a blender, combine raspberries, vanilla protein powder, lemon zest, lemon juice, coconut water, and agave nectar.

2. Blend until smooth.

3. Transfer the mixture into a freezer-safe container and freeze for at least 5 hours.

4. Allow the sorbet to thaw for a few minutes before serving.

Nutritional Info (per serving): Calories: 130 Protein: 8g (23%) Carbohydrate: 18g (46%) Fat: 2g (15%) Sodium: 20mg Potassium: 280mg Fiber: 6g

Peanut Butter Banana Protein Ice Pops

Satisfy your cravings with these creamy and protein-rich Peanut Butter Banana Ice Pops, a deliciously wholesome frozen treat.

Preparation Time: 15 minutes
Freezing Time: 4 hours
Total Time: 4 hours 15 minutes
Serving Size: 1 ice pop

Ingredients:

2 ripe bananas
1/2 cup vanilla protein powder
2 tablespoons natural peanut butter
1 cup unsweetened almond milk
1 tablespoon honey (optional)

Directions:

1. In a blender, combine ripe bananas, vanilla protein powder, peanut butter, almond milk, and honey.
2. Blend until smooth.
3. Pour the mixture into ice pop molds and freeze for at least 4 hours.
4. Run molds under warm water to release the ice pops.

Nutritional Info (per serving): Calories: 190 Protein: 15g (31%) Carbohydrate: 22g (42%) Fat: 7g (27%) Sodium: 70mg Potassium: 430mg Fiber: 4g

Vanilla Almond Protein Smoothie

Enjoy a delicious and protein-packed smoothie with the classic combination of vanilla and almonds.

Preparation Time: 5 minutes
Total Time: 5 minutes
Serving Size: 1 smoothie

Ingredients:

1 cup unsweetened almond milk
1/2 cup vanilla protein powder
1 tablespoon almond butter
1 teaspoon vanilla extract
Ice cubes (optional)

Directions:

1. In a blender, combine almond milk, vanilla protein powder, almond butter, and vanilla extract.

2. Blend until mixture is smooth.
3. Add ice cubes and blend again if needed.
4. Pour into a glass and enjoy this protein-rich vanilla almond delight.
Nutritional Info (per serving): Calories: 220 Protein: 25g (45%) Carbohydrate: 5g (9%) Fat: 11g (46%) Sodium: 180mg Potassium: 280mg Fiber: 2g

Berry Protein Smoothie Bowl

Start your day with a vibrant and nutrient-packed Berry Protein Smoothie Bowl. It's a delicious and visually appealing way to enjoy a high-protein breakfast.

Preparation Time: 10 minutes

Total Time: 10 minutes

Serving Size: 1 bowl

Ingredients:

1 cup mixed berries (strawberries, blueberries, raspberries)

1/2 cup vanilla protein powder

1/2 cup unsweetened almond milk

1 ripe banana, frozen

Toppings: sliced almonds, chia seeds, fresh berries

Directions:

1. In a blender, combine mixed berries, vanilla protein powder, almond milk, and frozen banana.

2. Blend until smooth and thick.

3. Pour the smoothie into a bowl.

4. Top with sliced almonds, chia seeds, and fresh berries.

5. Enjoy this protein-rich and visually appealing smoothie bowl.

Nutritional Info (per serving): Calories: 280 Protein: 30g (43%) Carbohydrate: 30g (43%) Fat: 5g (14%) Sodium: 90mg Potassium: 470mg Fiber: 8g

Matcha Protein Iced Latte

Experience the unique flavor of matcha in a protein-packed iced latte. It's a refreshing and energizing beverage.
Preparation Time: 8 minutes
Total Time: 8 minutes
Serving Size: 1 latte
Ingredients:
1 teaspoon matcha powder
1/2 cup hot water
1/2 cup unsweetened almond milk
1/2 cup vanilla protein powder
Ice cubes
Optional: sweetener of choice (stevia, agave, or maple syrup)
Directions:
1. In a bowl, whisk matcha powder with hot water until frothy.
2. In a separate container, mix almond milk with vanilla protein powder.
3. Pour the matcha mixture over ice cubes.
4. Gently pour the protein-infused almond milk over the matcha.
5. If desired, add sweetener to taste and stir.
6. Enjoy this refreshing Matcha Protein Iced Latte.
Nutritional Info (per serving):Calories: 160 Protein: 20g (50%) Carbohydrate: 5g (12%) Fat: 7g (32%) Sodium: 180mg Potassium: 200mg Fiber: 2g

Chocolate Avocado Protein Smoothie

Indulge in a rich and creamy chocolate smoothie packed with the goodness of avocado and protein.
Preparation Time: 8 minutes
Total Time: 8 minutes
Serving Size: 1 smoothie
Ingredients:
1/2 avocado
1 cup unsweetened almond milk
1/4 cup chocolate protein powder
1 tablespoon unsweetened cocoa powder
Ice cubes
Optional: sweetener of choice (stevia, agave, or maple syrup)
Directions:

1. In a blender, combine avocado, almond milk, chocolate protein powder, and cocoa powder.
2. Add the ice cubes to the blender and blend until smooth.
3. If desired, add sweetener to taste and blend again.
Pour into a glass and enjoy this chocolatey, protein-packed treat.
Nutritional Info (per serving): Calories: 250 Protein: 20g (32%) Carbohydrate: 15g (24%) Fat: 15g (44%) Sodium: 150mg Potassium: 550mg Fiber: 7g

Peanut Butter Banana Protein Shake

Satisfy your cravings with the classic combination of peanut butter and banana in a protein-rich shake.
Preparation Time: 5 minutes
Total Time: 5 minutes
Serving Size: 1 shake
Ingredients:
1 ripe banana
1 cup unsweetened almond milk
1/4 cup vanilla protein powder
2 tablespoons natural peanut butter
Ice cubes
Directions:
1. In a blender, combine banana, almond milk, vanilla protein powder, and peanut butter.
2. Add ice cubes to the blender and blend until smooth.
3. Pour into a glass and relish this delicious Peanut Butter Banana Protein Shake.
Nutritional Info (per serving): Calories: 300 Protein: 25g (33%) Carbohydrate: 30g (40%) Potassium: 550mg Fiber: 5g

Strawberry Basil Protein Infusion

Elevate your hydration with this refreshing Strawberry Basil Protein Infusion, a unique twist on a classic drink.
Preparation Time: 10 minutes
Total Time: 10 minutes
Serving Size: 1 glass
Ingredients:
1 cup fresh strawberries, hulled and sliced
1/2 cup fresh basil leaves
1 cup cold water

1/4 cup vanilla protein powder
Ice cubes
Optional: sweetener of choice (stevia, agave, or honey)
Directions:
1. In a pitcher, combine strawberries, basil leaves, and cold water.
2. Allow the mixture to infuse for about 1 hour in the refrigerator.
3. Strain the infused water into a glass.
4. In a separate bowl, mix vanilla protein powder with a small amount of water to create a smooth paste.
5. Add the protein paste to the infused water, stirring well.
6. Add ice cubes and sweetener if desired. Stir again.
7. Enjoy this unique and hydrating Strawberry Basil Protein Infusion.
Nutritional Info (per serving): Calories: 90 Protein: 10g (44%) Carbohydrate: 10g (40%) Fat: 1g (16%) Sodium: 30mg Potassium: 300mg Fiber: 2g

Coffee Protein Smoothie

Energize your day with the perfect blend of coffee and protein in this delightful smoothie.
Preparation Time: 8 minutes
Total Time: 8 minutes
Serving Size: 1 smoothie
Ingredients:
1 cup brewed and chilled coffee
1/2 cup unsweetened almond milk
1/4 cup vanilla protein powder
1 ripe banana
Ice cubes
Optional: sweetener of choice (stevia, agave, or maple syrup)
Directions:
1. In a blender, combine brewed and chilled coffee, almond milk, vanilla protein powder, and ripe banana.
2. Add the ice cubes to the blender bowl and blend until smooth.
3. If desired, add sweetener to taste and blend again.
4. Transfer to a serving glass cup and enjoy immediately.
Nutritional Info (per serving): Calories: 180 Protein: 20g (44%) Carbohydrate: 20g (40%) Fat: 3g (16%) Sodium: 50mg Potassium: 380mg Fiber: 3g

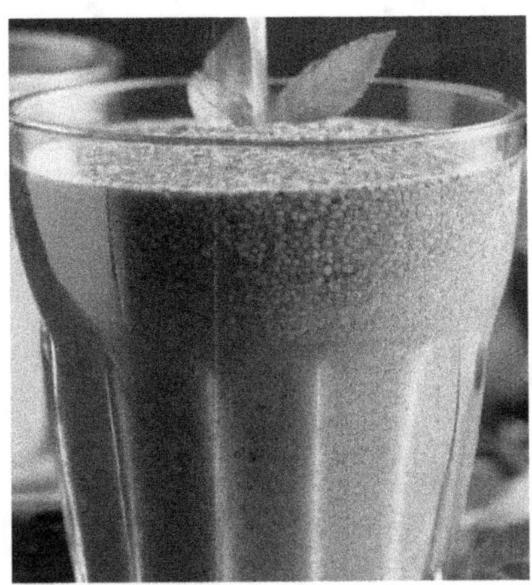

Cinnamon Chia Seed Protein Drink

Experience a delightful fusion of cinnamon and protein with this simple and nutritious chia seed drink.

Preparation Time: 5 minutes (+ 1 hour for chia seed gel)
Total Time: 1 hour 5 minutes
Serving Size: 1 drink

Ingredients:
1 cup unsweetened almond milk
1/4 cup vanilla protein powder
1 tablespoon chia seeds
1/2 teaspoon ground cinnamon
Ice cubes
Optional: sweetener of choice (stevia, agave, or honey)

Directions:
1. Mix chia seeds with 3 tablespoons of water and let it sit for about an hour until it forms a gel.
2. In a glass, combine almond milk, vanilla protein powder, chia seed gel, and ground cinnamon.
3. Stir well until the protein powder is fully dissolved.
4. Add ice cubes and sweetener if desired. Stir again.
5. Enjoy this nutritious and protein-packed Cinnamon Chia Seed Protein Drink.

Nutritional Info (per serving): Calories: 200 Protein: 18g (36%) Carbohydrate: 15g (30%) Fat: 8g (34%) Sodium: 160mg Potassium: 260mg Fiber: 7g

Mango Turmeric Protein Smoothie

Transport yourself to a tropical paradise with this exotic Mango Turmeric Protein Smoothie, rich in flavor and nutrients.

Preparation Time: 8 minutes

Total Time: 8 minutes

Serving Size: 1 smoothie

Ingredients:

1 cup fresh or frozen mango chunks

1/2 cup unsweetened coconut milk

1/4 cup vanilla protein powder

1/2 teaspoon ground turmeric

Ice cubes

Optional: sweetener of choice (stevia, agave, or maple syrup)

Directions:

1. In a blender, combine mango chunks, coconut milk, vanilla protein powder, and ground turmeric.

2. Add ice cubes and blend until smooth.

3. If desired, add sweetener to taste and blend again.

4. Pour into a glass and savor the tropical goodness of this Mango Turmeric Protein Smoothie.

Nutritional Info (per serving): Calories: 220 Protein: 20g (36%) Carbohydrate: 25g (45%) Fat: 5g (19%) Sodium: 40mg Potassium: 470mg Fiber: 4g

Green Protein Detox Smoothie

Revitalize your body with this nutrient-packed Green Protein Detox Smoothie, combining the power of leafy greens and protein.

Preparation Time: 10 minutes

Total Time: 10 minutes

Serving Size: 1 smoothie

Ingredients:

1 cup kale or spinach leaves

1/2 cucumber, peeled and sliced

1/2 cup unsweetened almond milk

1/4 cup vanilla protein powder

1/4 avocado

Juice of 1/2 lemon

Ice cubes

Directions:

1. In a blender, combine kale or spinach leaves, cucumber, almond milk, vanilla protein powder, avocado, and lemon juice.
2. Add ice cubes and blend until smooth.
3. Pour into a glass and enjoy the refreshing and detoxifying Green Protein Detox Smoothie.
Nutritional Info (per serving): Calories: 220 Protein: 25g (45%) Carbohydrate: 15g (27%) Fat: 10g (41%) Sodium: 150mg Potassium: 590mg Fiber: 7g

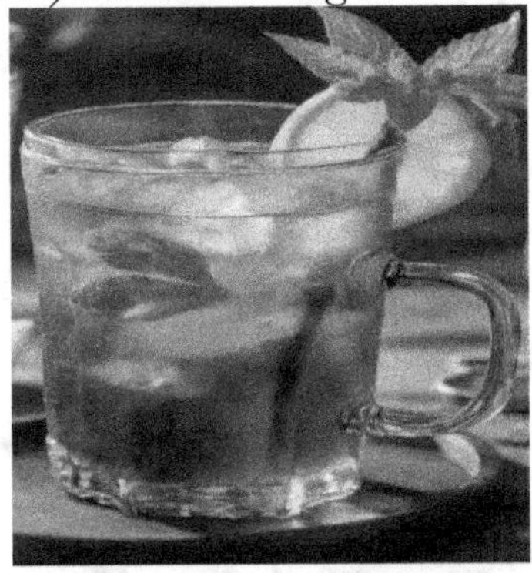

Protein-Infused Iced Herbal Tea

Stay cool and hydrated with this Protein-Infused Iced Herbal Tea, a refreshing beverage with a protein boost.

Preparation Time: 5 minutes (+ time to chill)
Total Time: 1 hour 5 minutes
Serving Size: 1 glass

Ingredients:
1 herbal tea bag (chamomile, peppermint, or your choice)
1 cup hot water
1/4 cup vanilla protein powder
Ice cubes
Optional: lemon slices, mint leaves, sweetener of choice

Directions:
1. Steep the herbal tea bag in hot water and let it cool to room temperature.
2. In a separate container, mix vanilla protein powder with a small amount of water to create a smooth paste.
3. Add the protein paste to the cooled herbal tea, stirring well.
4. Place the mixture in the refrigerator to chill for at least 1 hour.
5. Pour the chilled tea over ice cubes.
6. Garnish with lemon slices or mint leaves if desired.

7. Optional: add sweetener to taste.

8. Enjoy this protein-infused twist on a classic iced herbal tea.

Nutritional Info (per serving): Calories: 90 Protein: 15g (67%) Carbohydrate: 3g (13%) Fat: 1g (20%) Sodium: 40mg Potassium: 130mg Fiber: 1g

PROTEIN-PACKED BLISS BALLS RECIPES

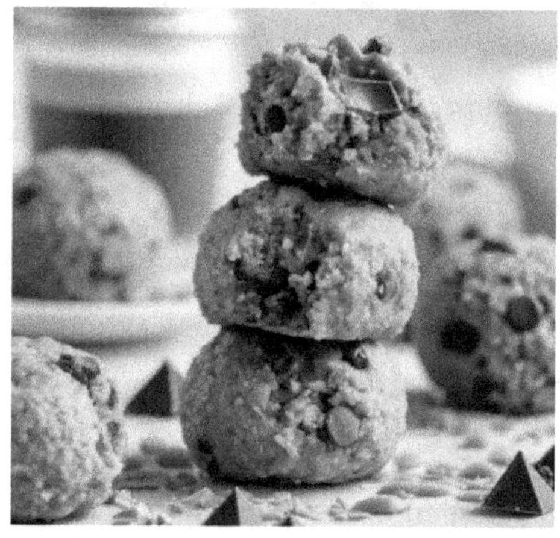

Almond Joy Protein Bliss Balls

Indulge in the rich flavors of coconut, almond, and chocolate with these Almond Joy Protein Bliss Balls. Packed with plant-based protein, these gluten-free, low-sugar treats are perfect for a guilt-free snack.

Preparation Time: 15 minutes

Chilling Time: 30 minutes

Total Time: 45 minutes

Serving Size: 12 bliss balls

Ingredients:

1 cup rolled oats

1/2 cup almond butter

1/4 cup chocolate protein powder

1/4 cup shredded coconut
2 tablespoons maple syrup
1 teaspoon vanilla extract
Pinch of salt
1/4 cup chopped almonds (for coating)
Directions:
1. In a food processor, combine rolled oats, almond butter, chocolate protein powder, shredded coconut, maple syrup, vanilla extract, and a pinch of salt.
2. Pulse until the mixture forms a dough-like consistency.
3. Scoop out small portions and roll into bite-sized balls.
4. Roll each ball in chopped almonds to coat.
5. Place the bliss balls on a parchment-lined tray and refrigerate for at least 30 minutes to set.
Nutritional Information (per bliss ball): Calories: 120 Protein: 6g (20%) Carbohydrate: 10g (33%) Fat: 7g (47%) Sodium: 15mg Potassium: 90mg Fiber: 2g

Peanut Butter Chocolate Chip Protein Bliss Balls

Satisfy your sweet tooth with these Peanut Butter Chocolate Chip Protein Bliss Balls. Packed with the classic combination of peanut butter and chocolate, these gluten-free, low-sugar treats are perfect for a quick energy boost.
Preparation Time: 15 minutes
Chilling Time: 30 minutes
 Total Time: 45 minutes
Serving Size: 12 bliss balls
Ingredients:
1 cup old-fashioned oats
1/2 cup peanut butter
1/4 cup chocolate protein powder
2 tablespoons honey or agave nectar
1 teaspoon vanilla extract
Pinch of salt
1/4 cup mini chocolate chips (for coating)
Directions:
1. In a food processor, combine oats, peanut butter, chocolate protein powder, honey, vanilla extract, and a pinch of salt.
2. Pulse until the mixture forms a dough-like consistency.
3. Fold in the mini chocolate chips.

4. Scoop out small portions and roll into bite-sized balls.
5. Roll each ball in additional chocolate chips to coat.
6. Place the bliss balls on a parchment-lined tray and refrigerate for at least 30 minutes to set.

Nutritional Information (per bliss ball): Calories: 130 Protein: 5g (15%) Carbohydrate: 12g (35%) Fat: 7g (38%) Sodium: 20mg Potassium: 80mg Fiber: 2g

Chia and Hemp Protein Power Balls

Elevate your snack game with these Chia and Hemp Protein Power Balls. Packed with nutrient-rich chia seeds and hemp protein, these gluten-free, low-sugar bliss balls are the perfect blend of health and indulgence.

Preparation Time: 15 minutes
Chilling Time: 30 minutes
Total Time: 45 minutes
Serving Size: 12 bliss balls

Ingredients:

1/2 cup chia seeds
1/2 cup hemp protein powder
1/4 cup almond butter
2 tablespoons honey or maple syrup
1 teaspoon vanilla extract
Pinch of salt
1/4 cup shredded coconut (for coating)

Directions:

1. In a bowl, combine chia seeds, hemp protein powder, almond butter, honey, vanilla extract, and a pinch of salt.
2. Mix until well combined.
3. Scoop out small portions and roll into bite-sized balls.
4. Roll each ball in shredded coconut to coat.
5. Place the bliss balls on a parchment-lined tray and refrigerate for at least 30 minutes to set.

Nutritional Information (per bliss ball): Calories: 90 Protein: 5g (22%) Carbohydrate: 7g (31%) Fat: 5g (47%) Sodium: 15mg Potassium: 80mg Fiber: 3g

Dark Chocolate Raspberry Protein Bliss Balls

Indulge in the decadence of Dark Chocolate Raspberry Protein Bliss Balls. These gluten-free, low-sugar treats combine the richness of dark chocolate with the tartness of raspberries, creating a delightful and protein-packed snack.

Preparation Time: 15 minutes
Chilling Time: 30 minutes
Total Time: 45 minutes
Serving Size: 12 bliss balls

Ingredients:

1 cup freeze-dried raspberries

1/2 cup chocolate protein powder
1/4 cup almond butter
2 tablespoons maple syrup
1 teaspoon vanilla extract
Pinch of salt
1/4 cup dark chocolate chips (for coating)
Directions:
1. In a food processor, pulse freeze-dried raspberries until they form a powder.
2. Add chocolate protein powder, almond butter, maple syrup, vanilla extract, and a pinch of salt. Pulse until well combined.
3. Scoop out small portions and roll into bite-sized balls.
4. Melt dark chocolate chips in a microwave-safe bowl.
5. Dip each bliss ball into the melted chocolate to coat.
6. Place the coated bliss balls on a parchment-lined tray and refrigerate for at least 30 minutes to set.
Nutritional Information (per bliss ball): Calories: 110 Protein: 5g (18%) Carbohydrate: 10g (34%) Fat: 6g (46%) Sodium: 10mg Potassium: 90mg Fiber: 2.5g

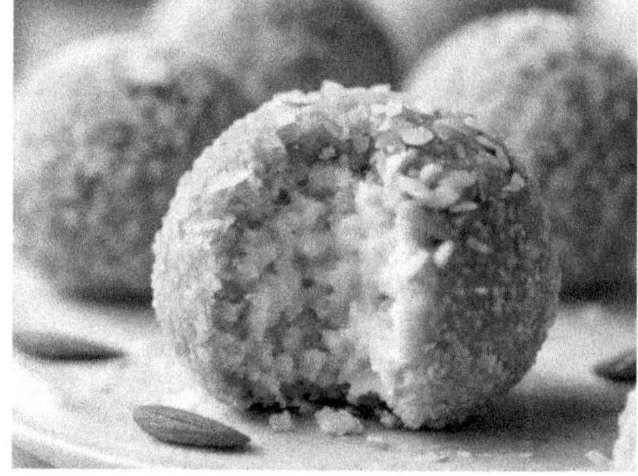

Vanilla Almond Protein Bliss Balls

Experience the sweet simplicity of Vanilla Almond Protein Bliss Balls. These gluten-free, low-sugar treats are enriched with the natural flavors of vanilla and almond, creating a delightful and protein-packed snack.

Preparation Time: 15 minutes
Chilling Time: 30 minutes
Total Time: 45 minutes
 Serving Size: 12 bliss balls
Ingredients:

1 cup almond flour
1/2 cup vanilla protein powder
1/4 cup almond butter
2 tablespoons honey or agave nectar
1 teaspoon vanilla extract
Pinch of salt
1/4 cup sliced almonds (for coating)
Directions:
1. In a bowl, combine almond flour, vanilla protein powder, almond butter, honey, vanilla extract, and a pinch of salt.
2. Mix until well combined.
3. Scoop out small portions and roll into bite-sized balls.
4. Roll each ball in sliced almonds to coat.
5. Place the bliss balls on a parchment-lined tray and refrigerate for at least 30 minutes to set.
Nutritional Information (per bliss ball): Calories: 90 Protein: 4g (16%) Carbohydrate: 5g (23%) Fat: 6g (61%) Sodium: 10mg Potassium: 70mg Fiber: 2g

Cinnamon Walnut Protein Bliss Balls

Warm up your taste buds with the comforting flavors of Cinnamon Walnut Protein Bliss Balls. These gluten-free, low-sugar treats are loaded with protein and the heartwarming essence of cinnamon and walnuts.
Preparation Time: 15 minutes
Chilling Time: 30 minutes
Total Time: 45 minutes
Serving Size: 12 bliss balls
Ingredients:
1 cup walnuts
1/2 cup vanilla protein powder
1/4 cup almond butter
2 tablespoons maple syrup
1 teaspoon ground cinnamon
Pinch of salt
1/4 cup crushed walnuts (for coating)
Directions:
1. In a food processor, pulse walnuts until they form a coarse meal.

2. Add vanilla protein powder, almond butter, maple syrup, ground cinnamon, and a pinch of salt. Pulse until well combined.
3. Scoop out small portions and roll into bite-sized balls.
4. Roll each ball in crushed walnuts to coat.
5. Place the bliss balls on a parchment-lined tray and refrigerate for at least 30 minutes to set.
Nutritional Information (per bliss ball): Calories: 110 Protein: 5g (18%) Carbohydrate: 5g (22%) Fat: 8g (60%) Sodium: 5mg Potassium: 70mg Fiber: 1.5g

Coconut Matcha Protein Bliss Balls

Experience a taste of Zen with these Coconut Matcha Protein Bliss Balls. These gluten-free, low-sugar treats combine the earthy notes of matcha with the tropical sweetness of coconut for a perfectly balanced snack.

Preparation Time: 15 minutes
Chilling Time: 30 minutes
Total Time: 45 minutes
Serving Size: 12 bliss balls

Ingredients:

1 cup shredded coconut (plus extra for coating)
1/2 cup vanilla protein powder
1/4 cup almond butter
2 tablespoons honey or agave nectar
1 teaspoon matcha powder
Pinch of salt

Directions:

1. In a food processor, combine shredded coconut, vanilla protein powder, almond butter, honey, matcha powder, and a pinch of salt.
2. Pulse until the mixture forms a dough-like consistency.
3. Scoop out small portions and roll into bite-sized balls.
4. Roll each ball in additional shredded coconut to coat.
5. Place the bliss balls on a parchment-lined tray and refrigerate for at least 30 minutes to set.
Nutritional Information (per bliss ball): Calories: 100 Protein: 4g (16%) Carbohydrate: 7g (29%) Fat: 7g (55%) Sodium: 15mg Potassium: 60mg Fiber: 2g

Blueberry Almond Protein Bliss Balls

Delight your senses with the fruity goodness of Blueberry Almond Protein Bliss Balls. These gluten-free, low-sugar treats are bursting with the sweetness of blueberries and the crunch of almonds, creating a perfect snack for any occasion.

Preparation Time: 15 minutes

Chilling Time 30 minutes

Total Time: 45 minutes

Serving Size: 12 bliss balls

Ingredients:

1 cup dried blueberries

1/2 cup vanilla protein powder

1/4 cup almond butter

2 tablespoons honey or agave nectar

1/4 cup almond meal

Pinch of salt

1/4 cup finely chopped almonds (for coating)

Directions:

1. In a food processor, pulse dried blueberries until they are finely chopped.

2. Add vanilla protein powder, almond butter, honey, almond meal, and a pinch of salt. Pulse until well combined.

3. Scoop out small portions and roll into bite-sized balls.

4. Roll each ball in finely chopped almonds to coat.

5. Place the bliss balls on a parchment-lined tray and refrigerate for at least 30 minutes to set.

Nutritional Information (per bliss ball): Calories: 90 Protein: 3g (13%) Carbohydrate: 12g (53%) Fat: 4g (38%) Sodium: 10mg Potassium: 50mg Fiber: 2g

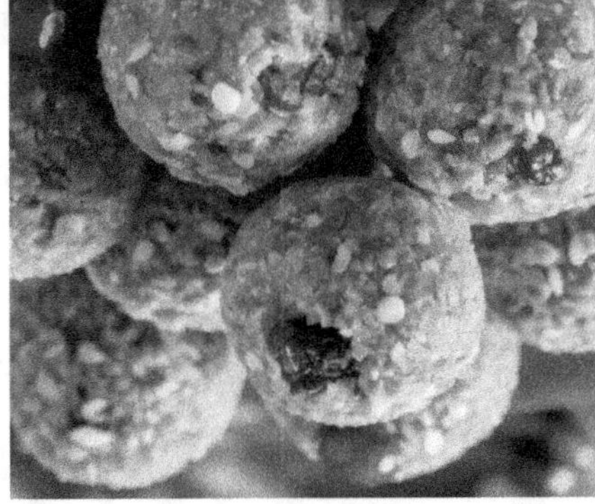

Cranberry Walnut Protein Bliss Balls

Experience a burst of tartness and nuttiness with these Cranberry Walnut Protein Bliss Balls. These gluten-free, low-sugar treats are enriched with the flavors of cranberries and walnuts, making them a delicious and satisfying snack.

Preparation Time: 15 minutes
 Chilling Time: 30 minutes
Total Time: 45 minutes
Serving Size: 12 bliss balls

Ingredients:

1 cup dried cranberries
1/2 cup vanilla protein powder
1/4 cup almond butter
2 tablespoons honey or agave nectar
1/4 cup chopped walnuts
Pinch of salt
1/4 cup desiccated coconut (for coating)

Directions:

1. In a food processor, pulse dried cranberries until they are finely chopped.
2. Add vanilla protein powder, almond butter, honey, chopped walnuts, and a pinch of salt. Pulse until well combined.
3. Scoop out small portions and roll into bite-sized balls.
4. Roll each ball in desiccated coconut to coat.
5. Place the bliss balls on a parchment-lined tray and refrigerate for at least 30 minutes to set.

Nutritional Information (per bliss ball): Calories: 100 Protein: 3.5g (14%) Carbohydrate: 15g (58%) Fat: 4g (38%) Sodium: 5mg Potassium: 40mg Fiber: 2g

Mocha Hazelnut Protein Bliss Balls

Indulge in the rich and aromatic combination of coffee and hazelnuts with these Mocha Hazelnut Protein Bliss Balls. These gluten-free, low-sugar treats are perfect for those who crave a delightful coffee-infused snack.

Preparation Time: 15 minutes
Chilling Time: 30 minutes
Total Time: 45 minutes
Serving Size: 12 bliss balls

Ingredients:

1 cup hazelnuts
1/2 cup chocolate protein powder
2 tablespoons instant coffee granules
1/4 cup almond butter
2 tablespoons maple syrup
Pinch of salt
1/4 cup crushed hazelnuts (for coating)
Directions:
1. In a food processor, pulse hazelnuts until they form a coarse meal.
2. Add chocolate protein powder, instant coffee granules, almond butter, maple syrup, and a pinch of salt. Pulse until well combined.
3. Scoop out small portions and roll into bite-sized balls.
4. Roll each ball in crushed hazelnuts to coat.
5. Place the bliss balls on a parchment-lined tray and refrigerate for at least 30 minutes to set.
Nutritional Information (per bliss ball): Calories: 110Protein: 5g (18%) Carbohydrate: 8g (31%) Fat: 7g (51%) Sodium: 5mg Potassium: 85mg Fiber: 2g